THE STORY OF VACCINATION

THE STORY OF VACCINATION

BY

Sarah R. Riedman

illustrated with 44 photographs

BAILEY BROTHERS & SWINFEN LTD
Folkestone

Published in Great Britain by
Bailey Brothers & Swinfen Ltd.
1974

SBN 561 00197 6

Printed in Great Britain by
Whitstable Litho Straker Brothers Ltd.

CONTENTS

ACKNOWLEDGMENTS

I am deeply indebted to Dr. R. J. Schnitzer, Director of Chemotherapy, Hoffmann-La Roche Inc., for his painstaking reading of the manuscript and his keen suggestions for alterations and revisions. Acknowledgment is most gratefully extended to Dr. A. J. Aeschlimann, Vice-President in Charge of Research, also of Hoffmann-La Roche, for his kindness in supplying and translating, from his library collection, the original of one of Paul Ehrlich's "blocks" (reproduced on page 161).

Heartfelt thanks are due to all the persons and organizations who have generously supplied the photographs that undoubtedly enhance this book for the young reader. These are: Dr. Louis Pasteur Vallery-Radot, grandson of Louis Pasteur, for his kind permission to reproduce the rare photographs from the family collection on pages 56, 59, 105; Mr. Milton Meltzer, Assistant Director of Public Relations of Chas. Pfizer & Co., Inc., for the loan of these photographs which were reproduced in the Pasteur Fermentation Centennial; French Embassy Press & Information Service for Frontispiece, and pictures on pages 44, 47, 53, 100, 107, 108, 124, 219; New York Academy of Medicine Photo-File for pictures on pages 13, 30, 33, 37, 68, 86, 111, 118, 121, 126, 129, 139, 148, 153; pictures from *The Story of Microbes* by Schatz and Riedman (Harper & Brothers) on pages 62, 82, 83, 136, 191, 193; British Information Services for the picture on page 64; New York Academy of Sciences for the picture on page 163; Antoni Gronowicz for pictures from *Béla Schick and the World of Children* (Abelard-Schuman, Ltd.) on pages 167, 179, 182, 184; National Foundation for Infantile Paralysis for pictures on pages 203, 209, 215; The Wellcome Historical Medical Library, London, for pictures from *Paul Ehrlich* by Martha Marquardt (Henry Schuman) on pages 132, 156; John Bale, Sons & Danielsson Ltd. (now Staples Printers Ltd.) London, for the picture on page 189.

S. R. R.

ILLUSTRATIONS

THE HUMAN TEST

FOR MONTHS the newspapers had been building up the story. This morning—it was April 12, 1955—the headlines were set; in fact, two sets were ready. Which ones would they use? No one had an inkling, although many tried to guess what the outcome of the study would be. The world held its breath awaiting the disclosure of the Big Secret.

It was the tenth anniversary of Franklin D. Roosevelt's death, and the men and women gathered in the auditorium of Rackham Hall on the University of Michigan campus had come to hear the results of the momentous experiment, one that had gone far beyond the confines of a university laboratory. Nearly two million children from 44 states took part in the test which had begun the year before, almost to the day. Hundreds of thousands of parents had given consent to have their children receive a series of three shots. Shots of what? Salk vaccine or a dummy? No one must know—not the parents, teachers, nurses, doctors, or health officials.

Vials, identical in appearance, had been coded, and the code would not be revealed until all the results were in. Six hundred and fifty thousand boys and girls between the ages of five and nine had lined up to bare their arms in clinics, schools, churches, and other public buildings. No one knew who drew the blank and who the active vaccine. Nearly twice as many Polio Pioneers in the same age group received neither. Yet they were just as necessary for the test. They were the "controls"—the group with which the others in the same towns and neighbourhoods would be compared.

For months information poured into the Polio Evaluation Centre in Michigan: vaccine lot numbers, ages, names, and locations of the children participants. Did any have reactions, and what kind? Did any develop paralysis? DID THE VACCINE WORK? Only when all the information was sifted, lined up, and examined would the answer be given.

On the morning of the 12th, the great field trial, largest in history and the mid-twentieth century way of tackling a problem in epidemic disease, had come to an end. Five hundred leading scientists and health officials, invited by the National Foundation for Infantile Paralysis, awaited the scientific judgment, along with other hundreds of newspaper reporters and radio, TV, and magazine writers.

How effective and safe had the Salk vaccine proved to be?

The last of the epidemic killers and cripplers—the poliomyelitis virus—was now all but conquered. Man had won another battle in the long war against his invisible enemies. The conquest of these scourges started more than two centuries ago, and the scientists who fought infectious disease are honoured heroes of the laboratory, bedside, hospital, and university. Our story is the story of their lives, adventures, hopes, and disappointments, their stumblings, mistakes, and lifesaving successes.

1

CENTURIES OF HALF MEASURES

"FUTURE NATIONS will know by history only that the loathsome smallpox has existed and by you has been extirpated." In these prophetic words, Thomas Jefferson paid tribute to Edward Jenner, the first of our heroes.

When Jenner was a boy, every tenth death in England was from smallpox. Nine out of ten persons who contracted it were children who had not yet reached their tenth birthday. Those who survived were left scarred; often they became blind, deaf, or even insane. Riches and fame were no protection. Nor did it matter on what continent or in what century one was born.

Louis XV of France and William II of Orange died of it. Beautiful Queen Maria Theresa of Austria didn't escape it, and George Washington was left with deeply pitted marks on his strong face. Centuries before that, this dreaded disease raged in China and India, among the Romans and Arabians. In Biblical Egypt "plagues of boils" broke out periodically. Some epidemics were mild, others dreadfully severe, and there was only one defence: those who survived one attack were protected against another. People knew this for as long as they knew of the ravages of repeated epidemics. If they let themselves contract the disease during a mild epidemic, they could escape it in its deadlier form, and a severe epidemic was almost certain to occur in their lifetime.

The Chinese people devised this method: they placed in the nostrils of a healthy person several dried crusts taken from the skin of a smallpox patient. They found that, with care, they could store the crusts in sealed vessels for months; the sick matter would retain its potency. Thus, they would "catch" the disease in a weakened form and obtain lifelong protection.

Lady Mary Wortley Montague, the beautiful wife of the British Ambassador to Turkey, learned another way to fight off smallpox. In 1717, during the reign of George I, she wrote to a friend in England: "I am going to tell you a thing that I am sure will make you wish yourself here. The smallpox, so fatal, and so general amongst us, is here entirely harmless by the invention of ingrafting. . . ." Women whose business it was to perform the operation would meet whole parties of people who sought inoculation. They carried a nutshell full of matter of "the best sort of smallpox." Making a little wound in the skin (the patient was free to pick the spot), enough poison to give the person a sample of the disease was inserted on the end of a needle.

So satisfied was Lady Montague with the safety of the procedure that she had her little son inoculated. Within a few days the boy was singing and playing, and couldn't wait until supper was ready, she wrote to her husband. For a number of years the noble lady used her powers of persuasion and her talent for letter writing to spread the practice to England. The embassy physician in Constantinople who witnessed the inoculation of the Montague household was directed by the King

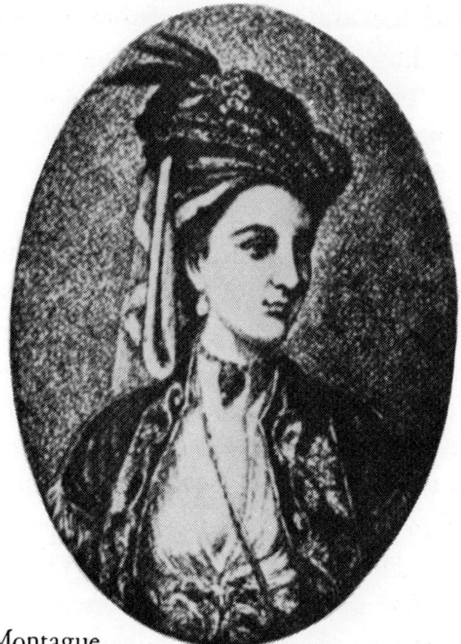

Lady Mary Wortley Montague

to try it on seven criminals condemned to death. They not only did well but thereby earned their pardons.

On her return to England, Lady Mary made some converts among doctors. One, Dr. Thomas Dimsdale of London, attained such a reputation with his inoculations that Frederick the Great of Prussia and the Crown Prince of Denmark had themselves inoculated by him. And the Empress Catherine of Russia invited him to spread the practice in her empire, rewarding him with a barony and a great fortune.

While this method, known as variolation or inoculation, was practiced widely in the Near East and the Orient for centuries, it was made popular in Europe chiefly through Lady Montague's crusading. But the very spread of inoculation kept the disease alive, for people not inoculated were always exposed to those who had it in the mild form.

The Arabs had a custom called "buying the smallpox." On the tenth or eleventh day of the disease, they squeezed a little of the sick matter from a child and introduced it into the skin of another. The patient was "paid" in candy, dates, or raisins. The "cure" often turned out to be as bad as the disease when another kind of infection set in. There were risks, to be sure, but that was the chance one had to take, although in France a law prohibiting the practice was passed in 1762.

Some were more successful than others in making inoculation safe. The apothecary Robert Sutton and his two sons set up an "Inoculation House" in Essex and made it a profitable business. It became a mecca where people flocked to be inoculated by the Suttonian method. The method itself was not really different, but Sutton took certain precautions in preparing the patient and in providing good care afterward. He prescribed a period of rest and proper diet to build up the patient, and just before the inoculation he gave a strong cathartic. He used only a small amount of the matter which he obtained from the blister rather than from the crust. By inserting the matter between the layers of the skin, he avoided drawing blood. By using only the upper part of the arm, which could be kept uncovered, he kept the inoculation spot clear of rubbing clothes. Avoiding dressings and bandages, he reduced the danger of infection. In fact, the precautions Sutton introduced to make variolation safer are still good today.

In America, inoculation was first introduced in 1721 by Zabdiel Boylston, a Boston doctor. He successfully inoculated his six-year-old son and two Negro servants. Several years later he described the process in a pamphlet which he dedicated to her Royal Highness, the Princess of Wales. When there was an accident, and a person died, inoculation of course received a setback. Then there were those who saw in inoculation the work of the devil. The practice defied the will of God, preached the Reverend Edmund Massey in Boston.

About the middle of the eighteenth century, Benjamin Franklin, then in England, interested himself in the subject. Together with William Heberden, a well-known London physician, he wrote a booklet on smallpox inoculation. Describing an epidemic in Boston which had spread to all corners of the city and temporarily cut it off from communication with the surrounding country, Franklin produced some statistics. Out of five thousand inhabitants who contracted the disease, about a thousand died, but of eleven hundred who had been inoculated only thirty died. "Notwithstanding the now uncontroverted success of Inoculation, it does not seem to make that progress among the common people in *America,* which at first was expected. *Scruples of conscience* weigh with many, concerning the lawfulness of the practice," he wrote.

Those who could hardly spare the high fees the surgeons charged for inoculation added to the hue and cry against the practice, and by teaching people how to do it, Franklin hoped to encourage parents to inoculate their own children. In the second part of the pamphlet, Dr. Heberden provided the "Plain Instructions" which were stripped of "medical terms and expressions used by physicians in their writings."

In the following two decades, American medical students who travelled to England and Scotland for their education brought back the Suttonian method of inoculation. Among them was Dr. Benjamin Rush, who enthusiastically promoted smallpox inoculations in Philadelphia, and credited the new method with building his early practice. As a surgeon in Washington's Continental Army he introduced inoculation among the Revolutionary troops, saving many lives. Before that, many more colonial defenders had died from smallpox than from British gunfire.

Like others in his day, Jenner went through the ordeal of "preparation for inoculation," which was recorded in the annals of his birthplace.

"He was a fine ruddy boy and, at eight years of age, was, with many others, put under a preparatory process for inoculation with the smallpox. This preparation lasted for six weeks. He was bled to ascertain whether his blood was fine; was purged repeatedly, till he became emaciated and feeble; was kept on a very low diet . . . and dosed with a diet-drink to sweeten the blood. After this barbarism of human veterinary practice, he was removed to one of the usual inoculation stables, and haltered up with others, in a terrible state of disease."

2

THE FIRST SUCCESSFUL TRY

Edward Jenner (1749–1823)

EDWARD JENNER was born in Berkeley, Gloucestershire, in 1749. If he had picked his birthplace, Edward probably couldn't have chosen a more beautiful bit of old England than the ancient market town in the valley of the Severn River. Poets have immortalized the charm of "Glos," as the people affectionately referred to Gloucestershire, one of the finest farming counties in all England. Gently rising from the green, luscious vale stood the low, treeless Cotswold hills. From the top of these could be seen the Berkeley Castle, where the Lords of Berkeley managed their feudal manor from as far back as Norman times in the twelfth century. And on a fair day one could see clear across the winding Severn as far as the Welsh mountains. Between the river and the mountains lay the rich dairy farms, apple and pear orchards, the heaths and hedgerows and clean villages with thatched roofs and rising church spires.

If Edward had prized social position he could have done no better than to be born into a family of clergy. On England's social ladder of that day, the Jenners occupied a very high rung, for members of the ministry of the official Church of England were held in high esteem. Reverend Stephen Jenner had received his master of arts degree from Oxford, and Edward's maternal grandfather, Reverend Henry Head, was once the keeper of the church funds in Bristol, an important port town some forty miles south of Berkeley. Edward was the third son. Following him were Mary, Sarah, and Ann. His oldest brother, bearing his father's name, became a clergyman as did Henry the next oldest, and Ann married a minister.

The Old Vicarage where his father was vicar and where Edward spent his boyhood years, was an imposing, rather grim, twin-gabled stone structure. Its enormous windows, sectioned into dozens of little panes, were set high above the ground. A stone wall enclosed the spacious grounds of the fine old country home. The pleasures of a country gentleman—riding, hunting, reading, and entertaining—were open to its inhabitants, who owed their livelihood to the Berkeleys, the main landholders of the area.

Edward was attached to his home, but perhaps the combination of a quiet, modest, friendly nature, love for rural life, and his profession later took him out of the austere seclusion of the vicarage and into the neighborhood of simple, friendly folk. But we are getting ahead of our story.

His father died when Edward was only five, and Stephen, considerably older than the rest of the children, took over the household tasks of vicar and head of the family. Apparently he did very well as guardian-father and capably looked after the family fortune. As was customary in those days, he taught the younger children at home and later selected their professions. George and Henry were to enter the church, and medicine was happily arranged for Edward when he was only thirteen.

Edward's formal schooling began when he was about eight

or nine. A short distance from Berkeley, in the village of Wotton-under-Edge, Reverend Mr. Clissold conducted a school for the sons of the upper crust of Gloucester folk. Besides religion, the education for a gentleman was heavily weighted on the side of the classics. Learning to read, write, and memorize Latin and Greek verse was an essential part of the curriculum and was started very early. If the fidgetiness of youth distracted the pupils from their studies, there were simple ways of enforcing attention. A closet full of canes of varying sizes to suit each degree of infraction of the rules kept the boys in line.

Edward made good progress in his school work, considering that he showed an early interest in natural science and that this had no place in the school curriculum. When he was nine, he made a collection of the nests of dormice—hibernating "mice" that look like squirrels. After he had exhausted the offerings of the village school and gone on to a larger one in Cirencester, his interest in fossils resulted in a fine collection dug out of nearby limestone.

When Edward was just entering his teens, he was apprenticed to Mr. Daniel Ludlow in the town of Chipping Sodbury, southeast of Berkeley, not far from Bristol. From Mr. Ludlow he was to learn the practical art of medicine and surgery. Few physicians received their training in a university medical school, but whether they did or not, all had to serve a long apprenticeship. A surgeon's apprentice lived in his master's home and shared the life of the family. He assisted in the dispensary and dressing room and accompanied his master on home calls. Here he learned to wield the scalpel, pound out the medicines with pestle and mortar, and weigh the ingredients on the dispensary scale.

By working hard for a number of years, an apprentice could learn as much as his master knew, and as soon as he could be trusted on his own, he was permitted to try his hand at the healing art. An apprentice's life was not easy because, in addition to cleaning up the surgery and instruments, his duties included running errands, bringing in firewood, and doing other household chores. In his spare time a zealous student could read the few medical books available, and perhaps try some remedies his master had never learned or had forgotten. Because of his bent for natural science and his warm sympathy for people, we can be pretty sure that Edward learned to observe and minister to the sick during his seven years' apprenticeship.

When he was twenty, he had the good fortune to go on to study with the famous Dr. John Hunter in London. Only a few names survive from each century in medical history. That of the Hunter brothers is among them. William Hunter, ten years older than John, was the pride of his family. He studied medicine in Glasgow, was a successful surgeon with a vast practice in London, taught anatomy to many celebrated doctors, and earned a reputation as an outstanding obstetrician.

John was dull at school and assisted his brother-in-law, who was a timber merchant, but his interests lay in other directions. He wanted to know all about clouds, grasses, and why leaves changed colour in the autumn. He watched ants, birds, bees, tadpoles, and worms, and pestered people with questions about them which they couldn't answer, and with which they were bored anyway. John persuaded William to take him on as an assistant in the school of anatomy he maintained in his home. The ne'er-do-well brother soon proved himself in his chosen work. William sent him to Oxford to make up his deficiencies in education, but he left after a few months with protests that they wanted to make an old woman of him, "stuffing" him with Latin. Proving to be one of those rare geniuses who shine without benefit of a university education, John eventually eclipsed his famous brother as a surgeon, anatomist, and experimental scientist.

John Hunter's contributions to medical science are numerous: he was the first to describe the development of the teeth, the tear ducts, the blood supply to the uterus, and surgical shock. His passion was collecting. There was a purpose to his wonderful collection and the strange menagerie he maintained in his home. Whether he studied the air-sacs of birds, electric organs of fish, the skeletons of whales and sea-cows, or the development of the ear membranes in the cow, deer, and hare, his interest was in the logical connection between similar structures. For he believed that in the early stages of their development, animals exhibited features that resembled those of simpler animals.

He spent most of his earnings as a surgeon on his collection, and willed it to the British Government, but during Hunter's lifetime, when he tried to sell it at a low price, the younger Pitt, who was then Prime Minister, said: "What! buy preparations! Why, I have not enough money to buy gunpowder!"

Edward Jenner's own love of nature was bound to flower in a school where the atmosphere was so favourable to scientific observation. He lived in the home of John Hunter, twenty years older than himself, but a kindred spirit. The two men became lifelong friends. When Jenner, after several years at formal study, took up the practice of his profession they exchanged not only letters but specimens. The master requested a "large porpoise, for love or money," young blackbirds of different ages, crows' and magpies' nests and a bustard, saying: "Dear Jenner, I do not know anyone I would sooner write to than you: I do not know anybody I am so much obligated to."

Together master and pupil investigated hibernation, finding

that the temperature of hedgehogs during winter sleep is the same as that of their frozen burrows, the heart beats only fourteen times a minute, and breathing is practically at a standstill. Is it only a step in the direction of hibernation when in the winter wrens sleep for the better part of the day, huddled together for warmth? Perhaps even primitive man slept through the winter months in the darkness of the cave where he put away a little food until life awakened in the spring.

Jenner could not have found a better school in which to nurture his interest in living things and to prepare himself for his profession. In turn, John Hunter was grateful for having a student after his own heart, an observer of nature.

But Edward had to keep up with his master's exacting and rigorous schedule. Hunter rose at six and dissected until breakfast at nine. By nine-thirty and until noon he was seeing patients in his office. Lunch was simple and brief, and he was off on calls and hospital rounds. After an early dinner he would sleep for an hour, and after that his time was "his own." Until midnight he experimented, read, wrote lectures, and made notes about his observations. No specimen was too far-fetched a subject for Dr. Hunter to scrutinize: it could be goose eggs for the study of embryology, pond water for fresh-water life, the skeleton of a giant bear contracted for with a travelling gypsy when it was still dancing, a rare bird or serpent.

In the most roundabout way, an animal experiment sometimes led to a new principle in human surgery. One time Dr. Hunter was studying the growth of antlers in deer. He found that if he tied off the artery to the head on one side the antler became cold, but in a few weeks the circulation was completely restored. When the deer died (not as a result of the operation), an autopsy showed that the blood had been shunted through other blood vessels.

Some time later a patient with a clot inside a large pocket of a stretched artery in the knee was admitted to the hospital in a serious condition. The customary treatment was to tie the vessel above and below the clot, and then scoop the clot out of the pocket. The procedure was fatal so often that amputation was considered safer. Hunter recalled the experiment with the deer's antler. He tied the large artery in the triangular space (Hunter's canal) between three muscles above the knee, shutting off that branch of the circulation. Within six weeks the patient was well, his leg having been nourished by the blood shunted from neighbouring connecting vessels. Since then the procedure has saved many a limb as well as life.

Jenner had the opportunity to learn not only from his illustrious master but from other celebrated physicians, botanists, and naturalists who crossed Hunter's path. Furthermore, London was the centre for many collections of specimens brought from all over the world. The newly opened British Museum housed a vast collection of treasures brought back by the young botanist Sir Joseph Banks, who had sailed with Captain Cook on his first voyage of circumnavigation. A valuable collection of specimens gathered by Linnaeus, the Swedish botanist, was brought to England by one of Hunter's pupils. The Linnean Society organized, and the Society of London Entomologists housed, a splendid collection of butterflies and moths.

Through Hunter, Jenner met Sir Joseph Banks. The collection brought back from his expedition needed to be put in order and when Banks asked Hunter for help, the latter recommended Jenner. The personable young student made such an agreeable impression because of his good humour as well as his good work, that Banks in turn recommended him as naturalist for Cook's second voyage. Still another offer came from Hunter —an invitation for Jenner to stay on as his assistant.

Besides rubbing elbows with the scientific elite, Jenner also had a pleasant social life in London. He loved music, had a pleasing voice, and enjoyed both singing and playing the flute. Many delightful evenings were spent in the Hunter home in part-singing and in the playing of flute and piano duets with Mrs. Hunter.

But when the time came for Jenner to make a decision, he was eager to leave London, which he found crowded, noisy, and smoky. He chose to return to the countryside he knew so well and loved, and turned down the opportunities which offered a different kind of adventure from the one for which he was destined as a country doctor in Gloucestershire.

In 1773 the young doctor was back in Berkeley, making his home with Stephen at the vicarage. Jenner's attachment to his native village and family was only part of what drew him to his home town. To the very marrow he was a country-bred man. The clean air, the hills and meadows, the rivers and woods held more attraction than the strange mysteries of far-off lands. He loved nothing better than to ride through the countryside, a willing friend at his side to share with him the beauty of the scenery.

Full of wonder to the keen observer was the night-flowering primrose that saved its honey during the day, and opened its petals after sunset, its nutritious fluid attracting the busily sucking moths. Sir Humphry Davy, chemist and inventor of the safety lamp for miners, saw the dunghill as useful only to the worm. But Jenner recognized its importance to people. About the common earthworm he told Davy: ". . . wherever they move, they leave a train of mucus behind them, which becomes manure to the plant . . . they act as the slug does, in furnishing materials for food to the vegetable kingdom; and under the surface, they break the stiff clods in pieces and . . . divide the soil."

Jenner was more at home with country people and the quiet, simple life of a rural community. An old-fashioned Berkeley fair in May "spread joy around for many a mile," and became a subject of one of his poems. The rosy milkmaid quit her pail, the thresher put aside his flail, the woodman his rugged chain; delighted children swarmed around the toy stalls. After making their annual purchases, village folk flocked around the shows which included Jenner's natural history collection.

Perhaps his sympathy with people, his gentle manner, common wisdom, and kindly disposition, as much as his excellent medical training (thanks to Dr. Hunter) endeared him to his patients. Sometimes because it was convenient, but more often out of concern for his patient, he would stay overnight at a patient's home. The next morning he might make other calls in the neighbourhood and return to the patient, if the crisis had not passed. This custom helped to make him a confidante and an advisor to the family in matters that were frequently not medical.

He soon became established, his practice flourished, and from the time he saved the first patient he operated on at the Gloucester Infirmary, his reputation as a surgeon was assured.

The life of a country doctor was not easy. One winter day when summoned to a patient, he rode for miles through a blizzard on the Cotswold hills. His face and neck wrapped in ice, the snow drifting under his hat, he arrived with his limbs all but numb. "When I came to the house I was unable to dismount without assistance. I was almost senseless, but I had just recollection enough to prevent the servants from bringing me to a fire." His discomfort gave way to the greater interest of the symptoms of exposure, and he went on to describe in detail the typical sensations.

Edward Gardner, an intimate friend, described Jenner as a "man intent and serious, and well prepared to meet the duties of his calling." He was well built, slightly on the stocky side, but robust and active. "Peculiarly neat," he dressed in a blue coat with yellow buttons, buckskins, well-polished boots with silver spurs, and carried a smart whip with a silver handle. He wore a broad-brimmed hat, under which his hair was dressed in the height of fashion—in a thick pigtail.

Jenner enjoyed the simple pleasures of neighbourly conversation, lusty glee club singing, violin playing, and versifying on familiar and homely themes, and had no regrets over his rejection of a career that might have brought him wider fame. There were times when his extensive practice took him to neighbouring towns—Rockhampton, Cheltenham, or even Bristol. He became an active member of local medical societies and met his colleagues in some member's home or at a favourite friendly inn. Over a pipe and a glass of ale they would read and discuss professional papers, and end the meeting with a meal of cold roast fowl, slices of beef, and jelly.

His regular correspondence with Dr. Hunter covered their mutual interest in natural history and professional matters.

"I received yours, and was extremely happy to hear of your success in business," Hunter wrote. "I hope it will continue. I am obliged to you for thinking of me, especially in my natural history. I shall be glad of your observations on the cuckoo, and upon the breeding of toads: be as particular as you possibly can. If you can pick me up anything that is curious, and prepare it for me, do it, either in the flesh or fish way."

Giving Jenner requested advice on a patient, in the same letter, he recommended cold baths, gentle exercise, and morning riding for the young lady's general health. Then he suggested she might take some medicine extracted from bark and a poisonous herb.

Acknowledging receipt of the cuckoo's stomach, Hunter asked Jenner to collect the eggs and the nests as well. Interrupting the thought about the cuckoo, he remembered: "This evening, looking into my book of patients, to scratch out the name of one who has just paid me, . . . I saw a Mr. Mathews of Berkeley recommended by you as your friend. . . . He did not pay me."

As Jenner's practice grew, he took in his nephew Henry as an assistant, about whom he wrote to a friend: " . . . tho' his mind is stored with ideas and do him the greatest credit, yet his general appearance and manner is so very 'fifteenish,' that a poor mortal on the bed of sickness will hardly look up to him with that eye of confidence and hope that might safely be placed in him."

For some years a disappointment in love cast a shadow over Jenner's satisfying life as a country practitioner. The wealthy young lady whom he was about to marry suddenly changed her mind. Soulfully, the unhappy lover confided in Dr. Hunter. But the older man consoled as best he could, from his greater wisdom:

"I can easily conceive how you must feel, for you have two passions to cope with . . . that of being disappointed in love; and that of being defeated, but both will wear out, perhaps the first soonest . . ." he wrote, and abruptly went on to talk about the weight of hedgehogs in winter.

After the unhappy incident Jenner immersed himself in his work, remaining unmarried for ten years despite the fact that many a matron eyed him as an eligible match for her daughter. Not until he was thirty-nine did he marry. This was the occasion for his leaving his brother and taking his bride, Catherine Kingscote of Gloucestershire, to Chantry Cottage, near Berkeley where they made their life's home.

To Gardner he wrote:

"My place of residence, though unfinished, is extremely comfortable; . . . my life, dating from the month of march [when he was married] has been the happiest beyond all comparison I ever experienced; and I will take it upon me to aver (nay I would swear it) that if you could be lucky enough to connect yourself with a woman of such a disposition as kind fortune has, at last given to me, you will find a vast addition to your stock of happiness."

A year later (1789) their first child, Edward, was born, and John Hunter was godfather.

Some important discoveries appear to be sudden, like flashes. But more often they burst into bloom only after many years of careful nurturing—observing, experimenting, testing, and retesting. Jenner's familiarity with dairy farming, the chief occupation in his neighbourhood, led him to observe the contagious disease of cattle which the farmers called the "cowpox." Small red pimples erupted on the cow's udders; a little later these became watery blisters. Finally, the blisters dried, forming a scab, and when they dropped off, left a pitted scar.

Vaccinia, the medical name for this disease, was spread from cow to cow by way of the milker's hands. Often a whole herd would become infected, and if some of the infectious matter from the udder passed through a scratch in the skin, the milkmaid or dairyman became sick. A week or so later the milker had a slight fever and the pimples on his hands went through the same changes as those on the cow's udders.

People in dairying districts believed that an attack of cowpox protected the milker from smallpox, and so they made little effort to avoid it. In fact, princesses greatly envied milkmaids their smooth faces, as they naturally lived in fear of disfigurement of their own.

At the medical meetings, Jenner brought up the subject of this immunity of milkmaids to smallpox, but he never got very far with the doctors. Although they were all familiar with this common belief, they pooh poohed it as an old wives' tale, much as we would today if someone said that eating garlic would protect against the plague. Each of the learned doctors could recall an instance of a person who had had both cowpox *and* smallpox.

Still, there were isolated instances of people who vaccinated* their children with cowpox, and though they couldn't prove it, this was actually the reason why the children did not get smallpox. Benjamin Jesty, a farmer in Dorset, vaccinated his wife and two sons in 1774, when a severe epidemic of smallpox raged. When fifteen years later one of the sons was inoculated with smallpox, nothing happened to him. Mrs. Jesty didn't do so well, for she nearly lost her arm from an infection that followed the vaccination. But Jesty's kin were sufficiently impressed with his success to inscribe the fact on his tombstone

---

*Vaccination which comes from the word *vacca* (cow) and *vaccinia* (cowpox disease) is the correct word for injection with cowpox matter. Inoculation or variolation means protection with smallpox matter. Today we use the terms "vaccination" and "inoculation" interchangeably, but in Jenner's time, vaccination distinguished his method from the older one of inoculation with smallpox.

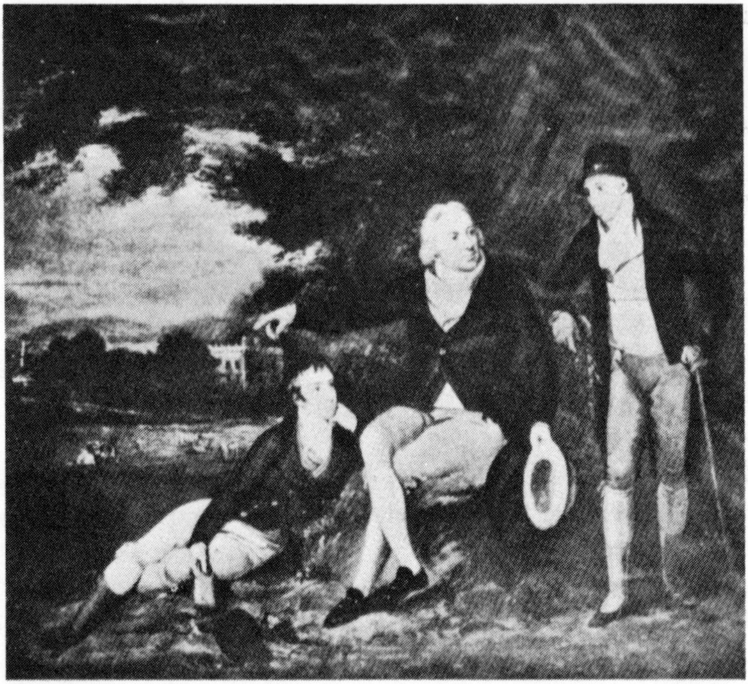

Dr. Jenner advises a farmer to use cowpox for vaccination

when he departed in 1816. But that was many years after the event which, at the time, nearly killed the practice of a doctor who suggested that Jesty's experiment might be tried on others.

It is hard to say when Jenner first became interested in the subject of vaccination, but it was certainly on his mind for many years. Very likely the thought first came to him when he was still an apprentice to Mr. Ludlow. A young girl who visited him as a patient, at the time of a smallpox scare, boasted that she was not afraid of catching the disease, because she had had the cowpox. Jenner recorded that this aroused his interest and that he put many questions to this girl.

Perhaps the memory of his own inoculation, which for

some time afterwards gave him nightmares and ringing ears, set him thinking about a way to improve upon the method.

When Jenner talked over the subject of vaccination with Hunter, his former master told him that the only way to find out for sure, was to make an actual test. "Don't *think,* Jenner, but try," he advised. Jenner himself wrote that he had investigated the subject for about twenty years. In 1789 he confided in Gardner; he thought he had found a way to eradicate the scourge of smallpox, but pledged him to secrecy: "I have entrusted a most important matter to you, which I firmly believe will prove of essential benefit to the human race . . . should anything untoward turn up in my experiments, I should be made, particularly by my medical brothers, the subject of ridicule, for I am the mark they all shoot at." By then he had been in practice for eight years, and had already studied the problem of vaccination long enough to earn the scorn of his colleagues. He would record every case of cowpox in the neighbourhood that he found conferred immunity to smallpox during an epidemic.

To his own observations he added notes of the experiences of other doctors whom he constantly plied with questions. But he had much less trouble collecting information from the farmers who strongly believed that an attack of cowpox made people safe against smallpox. A hired hand who had had cowpox had a better chance of a job than one who hadn't been so stricken. People who had contracted the milder disease were employed as nurses in an epidemic of smallpox. Jenner recounts the story of a matron who had accidentally taken cowpox through handling infected milk pails. Shortly afterwards the lady attended a relative who died from smallpox, but didn't herself get the disease.

As Jenner became more convinced, he went on to experiment. He inoculated with matter taken from smallpox pustules persons who he believed had become immunized by cowpox. They either failed to react at all, or were made only slightly sick from the procedure. But occasionally he met with disturbing exceptions that shook him. Why was it that some milkmaids who had had eruptions on their hands and should have been protected had succumbed to smallpox later? Why did not all cases of cowpox bring immunity?

As he pursued his observations he found that not all the eruptions on the cows' udders which the farmers called cowpox were the same. Jenner learned to separate what was true cowpox from other types of eruptions. This answered part of the question. But even when some people unquestionably had true cowpox they weren't always protected. After pondering over this for a long time, he came to the conclusion that the cowpox disease was sometimes weaker than at other times and therefore provided only partial immunity.

Jenner had no way of knowing how cowpox was started; incorrectly he believed that it came from a disease that affected the feet of horses, and that farm hands working with both horses and cattle carried the disease to the cattle. Much later it was shown that this disease in horses—"grease," as it was called locally—had nothing to do with cowpox. But Jenner could hardly know about the invisible cause of cowpox or smallpox, because it was considerably later when viruses were discovered.

When his son was barely a year old, Jenner was sufficiently convinced that the disease transferred from an animal would protect against smallpox, so he inoculated the baby with swinepox. A week later, a few pustules appeared, making the child somewhat irritable. Later Jenner inserted a bit of smallpox matter into scratches in the child's arm, but several trials brought no results. Two years later, in 1792, a repetition of the procedure caused considerable redness of the spot. The vaccination "took"—we would say today—but it was not yet complete proof.

For several years afterward, for some unexplained reason, there were almost no cases of cowpox on dairy farms. Besides, Jenner had fallen ill with typhus which nearly ended his life. His experiments were therefore delayed, but his concern with the subject never ceased.

In the spring of 1796, there was an outbreak of cowpox on a neighbouring farm. Sarah Nelmes, the dairymaid, became infected. She had stuck her finger with a thorn, and had a tiny scratch through which the diseased matter entered. Jenner seized his opportunity. He collected the matter from the pustule on Sarah's hand and vaccinated James Phipps, an eight-year-old boy. A few weeks later, he inoculated the child with fresh smallpox fluid taken from a blister. There was no reaction.

Writing to Gardner whom years before he had entrusted

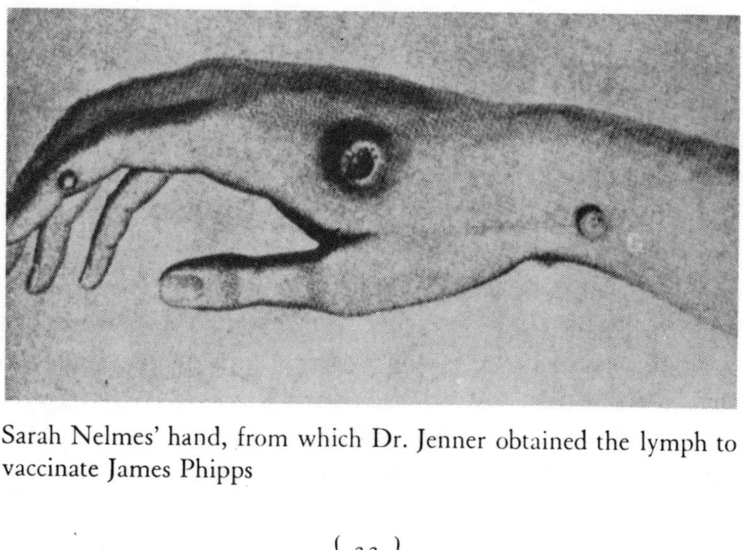

Sarah Nelmes' hand, from which Dr. Jenner obtained the lymph to vaccinate James Phipps

with his secret, he said: "A boy of the name of Phipps was inoculated in the arm from a pustule on the hand of a young woman who was infected by her master's cows . . . But now listen to the most delightful part of my story. The boy has since been inoculated for the smallpox which, as I ventured to predict, produced no effect. I shall now pursue my experiments with redoubled ardour."

He inoculated smallpox matter into ten persons who had at some previous time contracted cowpox. They too resisted smallpox. The evidence was complete. He was satisfied that he had put a vague belief on a scientific basis.

"I placed it on a rock where I knew it would be immovable before I invited the public to take a look at it," he said.

The elated Dr. Jenner was ready to make his great discovery known to the Royal Society. In 1796 he presented his results to the Society, but the paper was refused. A colleague urged him to enlarge on his findings by making further experiments, and then publish his results in a book. For the next two years the doctor collected more evidence, wrote, and revised, and finally was ready with a manuscript.

He and his wife travelled to London to demonstrate his discovery to the sceptical doctors in the big city, taking along the pile of manuscript papers for the printer, and a small amount of vaccine matter. His story was received coolly, and during the three months of his stay in London no one could be found who would submit to a demonstration of his discovery. Before returning to Berkeley, Jenner left, with a surgeon by the name of Henry Cline, a small quill dipped in a bit of smallpox matter, and he also left his manuscript with a London printer.

By that time the smallpox matter had become dry, but when a child with a tubercular hip joint came for treatment to

Mr. Cline, he reluctantly decided to vaccinate the patient over the joint. The surgeon's hope was that the inflammation in the skin would relieve the sick joint, just as a mustard plaster on the chest relieves a cold. In August 1798, the much surprised Mr. Cline wrote to Jenner:

"The cowpox experiment has succeeded admirably. The child sickened on the seventh day; and the fever, which was moderate, subsided on the eleventh day. The inflammation extended to about four inches diameter, and then gradually subsided . . . The ulcer was not large enough to contain a pea . . . I have inoculated him with smallpox matter in three places, which were slightly inflamed on the third day, and then subsided.

"Dr. Lister, who was formerly physician to the Smallpox Hospital, attended the child with me, and he is convinced that it is not possible to give him the smallpox.

"I think the substituting of cowpox poison for the smallpox promises to be one of the greatest improvements that has ever been made in medicine; for it is not only so safe in itself, but also does not endanger others by contagion . . ."

By that time the 75-page booklet containing Dr. Jenner's report had come off the press: *An Inquiry into the Causes and Effects of The Variolae Vaccine, A Disease Discovered in some of the western counties of England, particularly Gloucestershire, and known by the name of the Cowpox.*

Sir Benjamin Ward Richardson said about Jenner's booklet: "No book so small has been talked of so much: no book has been read from the original so little: no book of such dimension has made the name of any author so famous."

Finally the world knew that those who had cowpox were immune to smallpox; cowpox could be transmitted by vaccination; it gave the same protection as the disease itself. Vaccination with cowpox was not only effective; it was safer than the old method of inoculation with smallpox.

The Jenner vaccination was gaining acceptance, but not without opposition from those who had been practicing inoculation with smallpox. Some argued that children would become cow-faced, grow horns, and learn to moo rather than to talk. Cartoonists ridiculed the doctor-discoverer. Nor were doctors the least among the critics. Occasionally one, like Dr. Ingenhousz, would call attention to a failure—someone who had had cowpox and become a victim of smallpox. Dr. Jenner returned to London mainly to answer such doctors, but also to arrange for the publication of a follow-up pamphlet containing additional observations. He explained that those cases in which the vaccination didn't work were due to false rather than true cowpox.

Other obstacles stood in the way of complete acceptance of vaccination. The ignorant, and those less skilled than Jenner, who tried their hand at the new method, bungled. They failed to distinguish between true and false cowpox. Often they kept the matter too long or took it from old blisters, so that it had lost its effectiveness. If the puncture was too deep, there was danger of violent disease. The quacks neglected to follow Jenner's precautions to keep the fluid or *lymph* from the blister clean. Some squeezed the matter out of shirtsleeves stiffened with the discharge from blisters, selling the sleeves in strips. Frequently the lymph was contaminated, and made people sick. Those who failed jumped on Jenner, condemning vaccination.

But slowly Dr. Jenner was helping to overcome the difficulties. Pleas for vaccinia matter came from various parts of England, and even from other parts of Europe. As long as he could obtain cowpox lymph he sent it wherever it was needed. His nephew carried lymph to Oxfordshire where over 300 per-

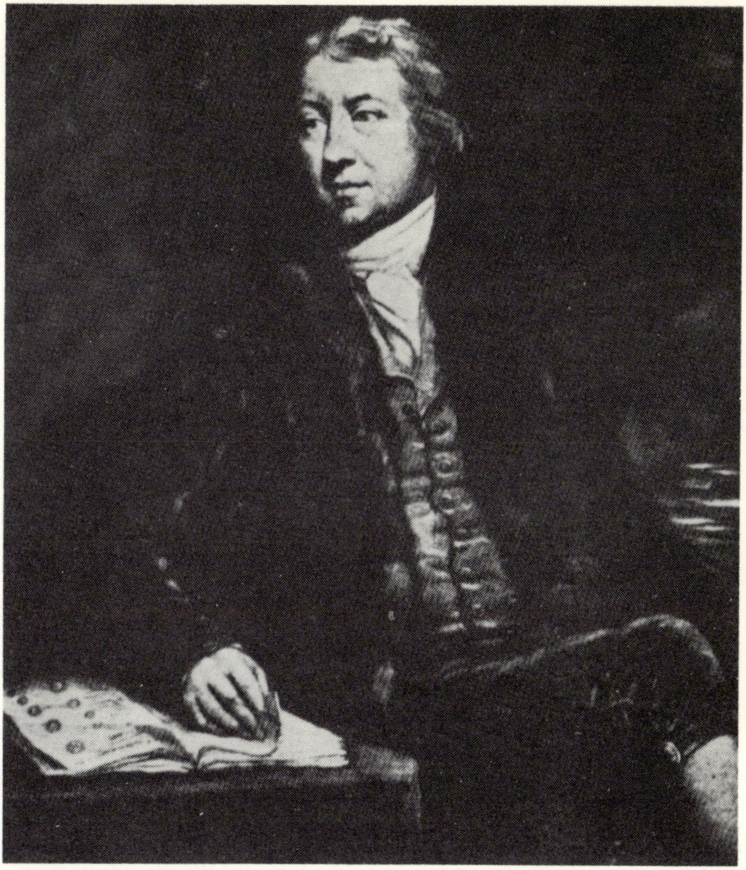

Dr. Edward Jenner

sons were vaccinated and afterwards more than half of these were inoculated with smallpox, as a test. They proved to be immune.

Jenner was offered 10,000 pounds a year if he would come to London to open an office, but once more the modest doctor turned down fortune and fame.

From all parts of the world came grateful testimonials,

money for Jenner to carry on the work of vaccination, announcements of his election to scientific societies. A temple was dedicated to him, and the Dowager-Empress of Russia sent Dr. Jenner a priceless diamond ring. The House of Commons voted a grant of 10,000 pounds. Lord Berkeley presented Jenner to the King and Queen and the Prince of Wales who wanted to know more about vaccination. But Dr. Jenner was much more gratified by the accounts of successful results, pouring in from everywhere, than by these many honours.

A severe epidemic of smallpox in Vienna in 1800 resulted in a desperate call for lymph with which to prevent future outbreaks. Doctors and sanitary officers vaccinated their children in Vienna and other cities, and the vaccine was sent as far as India. A doctor in Cambridge, Massachusetts, obtained the lymph for his children, and President Jefferson had his family and neighbours vaccinated. The British Government sent doctors to vaccinate the members of the fleet and garrison stationed at Gibraltar and Malta.

Sacrificing much of his practice, Dr. Jenner travelled to London to teach practitioners in the great metropolis the method of preparing and using the vaccine. Other nations sent representatives to England to learn the technique. Jenner spent much of his time answering letters from all parts of a clamoring world. He said of himself that he became "the vaccine clerk of the world." He used all his energies in his crusade to prevent the dreaded disease. A Jennerian Society was established and stations for giving vaccinations were opened in many places.

Reports of success poured in from far and wide. In Havana, where smallpox was nearly always fatal, there was no death from smallpox in two years; in Spanish America it was said to be extinguished. In France, out of two and a half million persons vaccinated only seven had taken smallpox. In Russia, 1,135,597 had been vaccinated in eight years. Since formerly every seventh child died each year of smallpox, "vaccination has saved the lives of 176,514 children in this Empire," the report read.

A meeting held by North American Indians sent word: "We shall not fail to teach our children to speak the name of Jenner, and to thank the Great Spirit for bestowing upon him so much wisdom, and so much benevolence. We send with this a belt, and a string of Wampum in token of our acceptance of your precious gift; and we beseech the Great Spirit to take care of you in this world and in the land of Spirits."

The country doctor became a public figure. Even Napoleon, at war with England, granted Jenner's request to release two prisoners of war, saying: "Jenner! Ah, we can refuse nothing to that man."

He also became a benefactor. The moneys that came in as grants from Parliament and other sources went in the same cause: for travelling, publishing, and assisting groups who would undertake public vaccination. Jenner once wrote to a friend who had guessed that he was getting rich:

"I know you fancy that the *cow* has fattened me, and that it is of no use to attempt altering your opinion. My domestication is the same now as it was before I cultivated her acquaintance so closely; except, that *then I had horses to my carriage,* and that *now I have none.* To know anything about me you should come down and inquire of my neighbours what I am, and what I was."

Jenner's last years were spent in poor health, sadness, and loneliness. His eldest son died in 1810 and his wife in 1815, both from tuberculosis. These personal tragedies saddened his old age, but did not keep him from his work. Every abuse, harassment from anti-vaccinationists, who misrepresented every accident and failure, only spurred him on in his mission to teach the correct method of vaccinating. As late as 1810, he wrote to a colleague: "Vaccination at its commencement fell into the hands of many who knew little more about it than its mere outline."

The day before he died he walked to a neighbouring village to arrange for the distribution of fuel to the poor. Returning from his charity calls in freezing weather he retired to bed. The next morning he had a stroke, his right side was paralyzed, and he died on the following day, January 26, 1823.

So ended the life of the modest country practitioner catapulted into immortality by his single-handed discovery which saved more lives than many a war had destroyed.

A century after the event, an American recently visiting in London was browsing through the *British Medical Journal* of 1858. He uncovered this strange story:

One hundred years after Jenner's birth a movement was started in England to erect a statue to the discoverer of vaccination. Doctors the world over gave generously to the fund. By 1858, when the statue was being readied for its unveiling, a debate was raging on the floor of Parliament. Was Trafalgar Square a suitable site? To be sure, Edward Jenner was "an ornament" to his profession, but was his statue as "eligible" as Lord Nelson's to stand in the Square that commemorates the battle of Trafalgar where Britain's greatest naval hero perished? Cowpox had its place, but surely not among the military heroes of the country, the Lords argued.

The editor of the *Journal* spoke for those who saw at least equal glory in shots without guns: ". . . we trust, in the name of national gratitude and common sense, that no more nonsense will be uttered against giving one of the greatest benefactors of mankind that place, which is of right his, among those who have deserved well of their country."

In the squabble over the site, the Lords apparently lost out, and one day in May 1858, Dr. Jenner's statue was inaugurated by His Royal Highness the Prince Consort. The *British Medical Journal* recorded that by permission of Her Most Gracious Majesty, the statue had been erected "on a most eligible site, in Trafalgar Square." There it stood for nearly four years until, no one knows how or why, it was moved. A brief news item on February 15, 1862 announced that "during the last few days the public have been surprised, on visiting Kensington Gardens, to find the statue of Dr. Jenner of smallpox vaccination celebrity . . . on a brand new pedestal," in London's lovely Kensington Gardens.

Pondering over the mystery of the removal of the statue, perhaps by the sabre-rattlers of that day, Borden S. Veeder who tells this story, comments: "The work of Jenner will be a living influence in years to come, when the name of Lord Nelson is but a dim figure of historic interest."

3

BUILDING ON BEDROCK

Louis Pasteur (1822–1895)

WITHOUT KNOWING why it worked, Edward Jenner found a way to protect people against smallpox. Everyone knew that the disease was somehow catching, but no one had the slightest inkling that it was microbes which caused infections. We skip almost a century and travel to France to meet the man who explained the ways of germs and how they produced disease.

It was 1854 when thirty-two-year-old Louis Pasteur was invited to be Professor of Chemistry and Dean of the School of Sciences at Lille. In the heart of the country of distilleries, this town in northern France would have seemed to offer little to a chemist who had already made a name for himself in the study of crystals. The very purpose for which this school had been established and paid for by the town was an innovation in French education. The young men who enrolled there were to prepare themselves for an industrial career. Some of the teaching methods were accordingly different from the traditional ones. For instance, in the universities of those days, experiments were demonstrated by the professor or his assistant. Pasteur, however, did not believe in demonstrations alone as a way of teaching. No science for science's sake for these students! In preparation for practical pursuits they would perform experiments *themselves.*

Pasteur welcomed the chance to put his knowledge to practical use. Doing his best to fire the imagination of his large audiences in the new faculty, he asked: "Where in your families will you find a young man whose curiosity and interest will not immediately be awakened when you put into his hands a potato, when with that potato he may produce sugar, with that sugar alcohol, with that alcohol ether and vinegar?" Imagine with what excitement a boy will tell his family around the dinner table that he has been working out an electric telegraph, he went on. Learning by doing is not easily forgotten. It is like learning geography by travelling. The boy who has analyzed the gases in air can never forget what it is that we all breathe, he continued.

It wasn't long before Pasteur, then thirty-four, happily married, established as a chemist, and looked up to by the gray-haired professors, was called on to work out a problem for the distillers. Had he been the kind of scientist who refused to "soil his hands" with practical questions, he might not have stumbled on the answer to an age-old problem. Its solution catapulted him into world prominence and immortality. What kind of man was he, and what about his early life?

The son of a tanner, Louis Pasteur was born in Dôle on December 27, 1822. His grandfather and great-grandfather had also been in the tanning trade. Having bought his freedom from serfdom by paying four gold pieces of twenty-four livres, Louis' great-grandfather went into the business of tanning leather. It was natural in those days for son and grandson

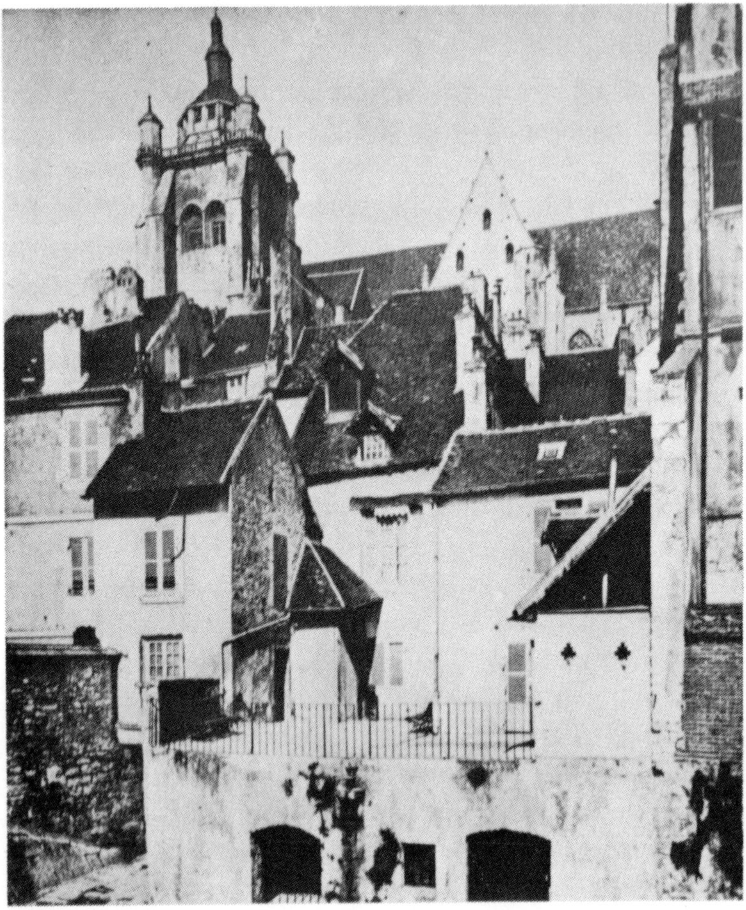

House in Dôle where Louis Pasteur was born, still in existence

to take up the same calling. But Jean Joseph Pasteur, Louis' father, must have dreamed that his only son (the third of five children) would have schooling—maybe even become a teacher in a small college!

Louis was too young to remember when his two younger

sisters arrived, or anything of his birthplace and the next house where his family lived for several years after he was born. The first of his memories was of his running around in the yard behind their small home in Arbois near the bridge that crosses the Cuisance River. Here his father had dug pits for steeping the skins that eventually were turned into leather.

M. Pasteur was a quiet, reserved man whose thoughts centered around his family. On Sundays when he donned his military-looking coat, adorned with the colourful ribbons of the Legion of Honour, one was reminded that the tanner was once a Sergeant-Major in Napoleon's Army. But he himself had long ago become resigned to the fate of a veteran of the lost Bonapartist cause led by the little man who by then had become a legendary figure. Jean Pasteur was now more concerned with the future of his children and especially his son's. When Louis was quite a little fellow his father taught him to draw, and the boy learned to handle crayons better than his father had ever done. In fact, he so much enjoyed making likenesses of his family and neighbours that he earned the name "artist," which was a source of worry to his anxious parents.

Louis was sent to the Ecole Primaire, the local school attached to the college of Arbois. The teacher divided his young pupils into groups, and appointed one of them monitor to help the others with reading and spelling. Louis, being the smallest in the class, had a great desire to become a monitor. And so he worked hard in his childish way but somehow he never shone. His teacher knew him as a plodder who achieved only average results. His father helped him with his lessons in the evenings, as much to learn as to teach the boy.

During holidays he could spend his time with his friends, especially with his dear friend Jules Vercel, net fishing in the river. But he would not join his companions in bird trapping, the sight of a wounded bird being not to his taste. He would rather invite his friends into the tannery yards for all its smells, where they could play with bits of bark and discarded hair scrapers.

No one would have said about Louis that he was "as smart as a whip" or "bright as a penny," but he was industrious in a way uncommon in children—he loved work. The principal of his school recognized this as something special in the boy. He also knew that M. Pasteur's ambition was to see his son become a teacher. And so he encouraged his pupil to prepare for the Ecole Normale in Paris, a school established by Napoleon to train young professors. The idea of their son's living alone in the great capital, separated from Arbois by two full days' journey, frightened the Pasteurs. But when an old Captain friend of the family and an officer in the Paris Municipal Guard promised to look after the boy, and even to get him into a preparatory school on a partial scholarship, they finally agreed to the principal's suggestion.

One rainy October morning, Louis, hardly sixteen, climbed on to the stagecoach. With him was Jules Vercel, also headed for Paris to study. The two were perched behind the coachman's seat trying to keep dry under a waterproof cover, as the elaborate preparations for the journey and the repeated goodbyes delayed the painful departure. Leaving his home and family was bad enough, but when at long last he arrived in Paris he was seized with painful homesickness. No matter how much he tried to hide his feelings from the boys and his teachers, his loneliness got the best of him. During his classes and sleepless nights he could think of nothing but Arbois. "If I could only get a whiff of the tanyard I should be cured," he told Jules Vercel.

After a few weeks M. Barbet, the headmaster, seeing the

boy's unhappiness, and fearing for his health, wrote to his parents. Then one morning a messenger arrived at the school, and with some mystery informed Louis that he was wanted at a nearby café. When the bewildered boy entered the shop he saw a man seated at a small table, holding his face in his hands. It was his father. No explanation was necessary. "I have come to fetch you," was all he said, and they were happily headed for home.

When the joy of homecoming had worn off, what was Louis to do? He was set adrift. He had no plans and so he turned to his favourite leisure occupation. With his coloured chalks he made portraits of everyone from the mayor to a pale little boy in a velvet suit. He returned to the school at Arbois where he

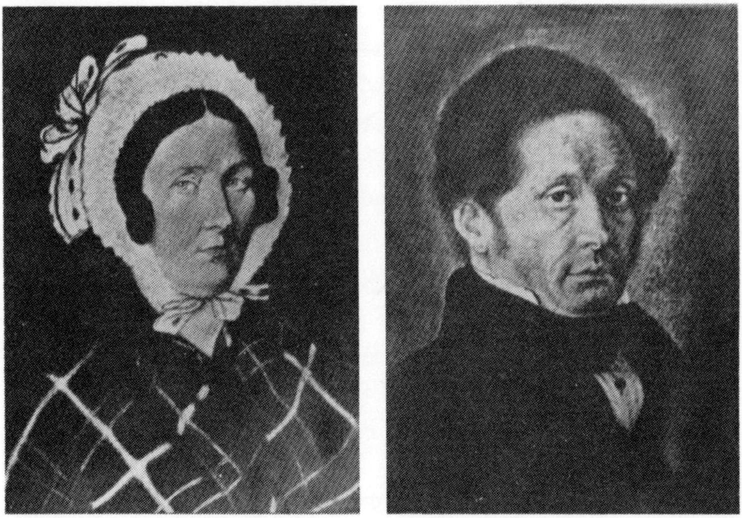

Photographs of portraits painted by Louis Pasteur of his mother (Jeanne Etiennette Roqui) and father (Jean Joseph Pasteur)

carried off nearly every prize, but he had outgrown the school by this time. Eventually, he determined, he would go to the Ecole Normale, but memories of his loneliness in Paris were still fresh. He decided to pass his baccalaureat at Besançon, a college about 30 miles from Arbois. His father's business brought him there several times a year to sell his tanned skins. In Besançon, Louis could prepare himself for the examination for the Ecole Normale.

Here he worked earnestly, and for the first time showed a wide-eyed curiosity in science. "With the aid of science one can rise above all competitors," he wrote home to his sisters. When he obtained his degree of Bachelor of Letters in 1840, his work was described as satisfactory in Greek, Latin, French, composition, medicine, philosophy, history, and geography, but very good in elementary chemistry. His earnestness, high sense of duty, and responsibility spoke more eloquently than his scholarly attainments, when the post of assistant master was offered to him at the college.

He carried out his monitorial duties ably and faithfully and satisfied the authorities; in addition he earned his keep and a small allowance. In the letters he wrote to his sisters, he tried to impress upon them the importance of work. "Will, Work, Success fill human existence," he wrote. "Will opens the door to success both brilliant and happy; Work passes these doors, and at the end of the journey Success comes to crown one's efforts. And so, my dear sisters, if your resolution is firm, your task, be it what it may, is already begun." Probably he used the same words when he addressed his young charges at the college.

The next year, as a supplementary instructor, his yearly salary was 300 francs, enough to enable him to get his own lodgings. He took on extra work, helping students prepare for the degree in science and mathematics. With the twenty or more francs he earned monthly from private lessons he offered to pay for his sister Josephine's tuition at a small college. But the suggestion from home was that he might better use this money to get private lessons for himself, to help him pass the entrance examinations to Ecole Normale.

The wisdom of his parents' advice was proven when, early in 1842, he was fifteenth of twenty-two eligibles for the examination. It was decided that he would have to keep on working hard at mathematics until the autumn. Once more he became a pupil in M. Barbet's school in Paris. In exchange for teaching the younger pupils from six to seven in the morning, he received a reduction of one-third of his fees. Living in a boarding school, he missed the privacy he had enjoyed in his own room at Besançon, but there were compensations.

The Barbet pupils had the privilege of attending classes at the Sorbonne, where the celebrated chemist J. B. Dumas lectured. His listeners were spellbound. "You cannot imagine the popularity of this course," Pasteur wrote. "The room is immense and always quite full. It is necessary to be there half an hour before the time to secure a good place, just as in a theatre." Here among six or seven hundred people at each lecture, a new world opened up for Pasteur.

His passion for accumulating facts, and his thirst for reasonable causes and proofs came to the fore. Now there was justification for his natural industry. It was foolish for his parents to worry about the temptations of the Latin Quarter. "When one wishes to keep straight, one can do so in this place as well as in any other," he assured them. "It is those who have no strength of will that succumb." In fact, Pasteur was hardly the sort of young man who got into scrapes. He spent his money frugally. He allowed himself two dinners a week at an inexpensive restaurant, occasional visits to the theatre and opera, with Charles Chappuis, a fellow student and close friend.

Finally, after a year in Paris, he got a first prize in physics, honourable mention in three other subjects, and was entered into the Ecole Normale, this time fourth on the list of applicants. Then came a brief holiday at Arbois, after which Pasteur was back in Paris several days before the other students arrived. On his first visit to M. Barbet, he offered to continue to help his boys in the physical science class.

The dilapidated and bleak building in which the Ecole Normale was housed had a grimness that fit in with the student's serious purpose. Jean Pasteur wrote to his son: "The details you give me on the way your work is directed please me very much; everything seems organized so as to produce distinguished scholars. Honour be to those who founded this School." At the same time, the anxious father wrote to Chappuis: "Do tell Louis not to work so much; it is not good to strain one's brain . . . Believe me, you are but poor philosophers if you do not know that one can be happy even as a poor professor in Arbois College."

How could M. Pasteur know how far his quiet, grave, but determined son would travel?

Study and research became Pasteur's complete existence. Always wanting to know more, to understand completely what he read and observed, he pursued his studies with a persistence that made any intrusion on his time unwelcome, even if Chappuis was the culprit. There was no better way to spend his Sundays and holidays than poring over a book in the library or in the laboratory, repeating some experiment demonstrated by Dumas.

One day Chappuis, acting on M. Pasteur's admonition not

to let his son work too hard, came to take Louis on some outing. Chappuis waited so long on a laboratory stool that he became reproachful; finally Pasteur took off his lab coat and half angrily said: "Well, let us go for a walk." But when they reached the street, Louis immediately turned to the inevitable subject of his reading, lectures, and experiments.

Chappuis' scholastic interests were in another direction. He was studying philosophy, and Pasteur's talk about certain quartz crystals that turned a beam of polarized light to the right and others to the left was to him just so much gibberish. But Pasteur had a gift for making things simple even to persons least inclined to understand them. His enthusiasm and his exhaustive reading of the history of any discovery soon made his listener feel that he was in on the story from its beginning. Chappuis found himself listening to the story of tartrate crystals which had been discovered, in the previous century, in the thick crust inside wine barrels—"tartar." But there seemed to be two kinds of tartrate crystals. Similar in form, and in the number and arrangement of their atoms, they behaved differently when examined with the aid of a reflected beam of light. One shifted the plane of light; the other, called racemic acid, had no effect—was neutral or inactive. Why? Many before Pasteur had been puzzled by this, and had worked over the problem, but as yet there was no answer.

If only he could devote all his time to solving this mystery! But he was preparing for his doctorate examinations and the problem of crystals was temporarily laid aside. After getting his Doctor of Science degree in 1847, he returned to his crystals.

Then came his first discovery. It dealt with the shape and structure of crystals. Some were built on a symmetrical plan, like the human body—each half was like the other. Others, like the human hand, could not be divided into symmetrical halves.

Pasteur noticed that the tartaric acid crystals had little facets on one half of the edge, but not on the other—they were asymmetrical. When he examined racemic acid he found *two* kinds of crystals—the facet of each tilted in opposite directions. They were, in fact, mirror images of each other, just like our right and left hands. Separating these out and then mixing an equal number of each of them again, he found that racemic acid did not turn the beam of light in his apparatus, while a solution of tartaric acid crystals did rotate the light beam. The shape of the crystals determined the behaviour of the solution! Some solutions turned the beam to the right, some to the left. But racemic acid, containing an equal mixture of both types, was inactive—the crystals of one neutralized the action of the other.

"I have it!" he shouted excitedly, rushing out of the laboratory, collaring the first person he met in the corridor and dragging him out to the Luxembourg Gardens. He had to tell someone of his discovery! Pasteur saw the "wonders hidden in crystallization, and, through it, the inmost construction of substances" which would one day be revealed, he said. On this discovery was built the branch of chemistry known as crystallography.

During the several years when Pasteur was making a name for himself in the realm of crystals he reluctantly accepted a teaching post first at the Dijon Lycée and then at the Strasbourg Academy instructing freshmen. Although he fulfilled his duties with his usual earnestness, his heart was in science. In a letter to M. Laurent, the Dean of the Strasbourg Academy, he confessed that "I can say no more than that, unless my tastes alter completely, I shall dedicate myself to researches in chemistry."

Pasteur's wife, Marie

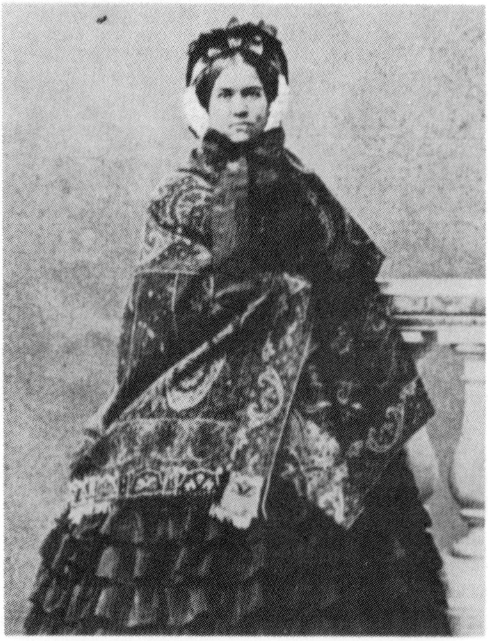

In this letter, he begged for the hand of pretty Marie Laurent, the Dean's daughter. When the reply was several weeks in reaching him, Pasteur, with sad resignation, wrote: "There is nothing in me to attract a young girl's fancy. I, who did so love my crystals!"

Finally, the proposal was accepted, and Louis and Marie were married on May 29, 1849. On the morning of his marriage the bridegroom was bending over his fascinating solutions in the laboratory, and had to be reminded that the assemblage was waiting for the ceremony. Soon afterwards, he wrote Chappuis: "I believe that I shall be very happy. Every quality I could wish for in a wife I find in her."

His home life did indeed turn out to be gloriously happy. Mme. Pasteur put her husband's scientific work ahead of everything. Sometimes she helped only by listening to explanations of his experiments, which somehow became clearer in his own mind as he talked about them. This usually happened when he was coming close to the answer to a problem with which he had been grappling. Other evenings she took notes from his dictation about his findings and the design of future experiments. His life work became hers also.

Pasteur was methodical and well disciplined. He planned his work so that he could do justice to his teaching, but at the same time save every possible moment for his research. "The nights seem too long for me, since I prepare my lectures without difficulty, and sometimes have five whole days a week that I can devote to the laboratory. I am sometimes scolded for this by Mme. Pasteur, but I comfort her by saying that I shall lead her to fame," he wrote to Chappuis.

Then came his two little girls who added to the joy and satisfaction of his domestic life. There was little to ruffle his peaceful existence in the early years of his career. He had accomplished enough to be respected by many of the older chemists and yet not enough to challenge their established beliefs. As yet he had made no enemies, because his work on crystals challenged no existing theory.

Just about the time when he came to the conclusion that the mirror-imaged tartaric acid crystals in the tartar of wine vats had something to do with the fermenting process, chance brought him to a place where he could study what goes on in brewing vessels.

In the summer of 1856, M. Bigo, a distiller of alcohol, brought his troubles to the young Dean shortly after he had settled in the School of Science in Lille. Bigo's son had studied in Pasteur's laboratory, but he came not as a parent. The beet-

Pasteur was investigating the vats at a bt. root fermentation factory. The bt. root juice didn't turn to alcohol & the industry was failing apart. He found that without yeasts present, fermentation wouldn't happen. But if rod-shaped bacteria were present, they produced acid that soured the beet juice. Thus he saved ailing bt. root industry.

root fermentation industry was falling apart. The beetroot juice in the vats just didn't turn to alcohol. Could M. Pasteur help? Pasteur grasped this opportunity of studying fermentation on a large scale. Hadn't he, in his classes, urged his students to make field visits to test out what they had learned in the laboratory?

The next day he was peering into the vats in the distillery, ladling out samples into little bottles to take back to his laboratory.

With a chemist's tools—the only ones he knew how to use —he found nothing that would explain why the murky mixture obtained from the "sick" vats contained no alcohol. For that matter, by chemical analysis of the healthy mixtures he got no nearer to answering M. Bigo's question. He would have to look at the fermenting juice through the microscope. With a little snare at the end of a wire he fished up a drop of the juice and placed it on a glass slide under his low-power lens.

He could hardly believe what he saw: teeming globules each encased in a wall. With his eye glued to his microscope he watched them change, "age," and finally sprout tiny buds. As he made careful drawings of these fascinating structures growing into chains which gradually broke apart, he wrote: "Before long the small bud, while still attached and joined to the large one, appears to acquire its own envelope and to be in itself an actual cell." Others before him had described yeast cells. This was no original discovery, but Pasteur didn't stop there.

When he examined a loop of juice from the soured vats he saw, in addition to these alcohol ferments, as he called the yeast cells, very short rods, single or in clusters. These were much smaller, hardly visible with the weak lens available to him. Still they were animalcules—living things. It was these ferments that produced the acid that soured the beet juice.

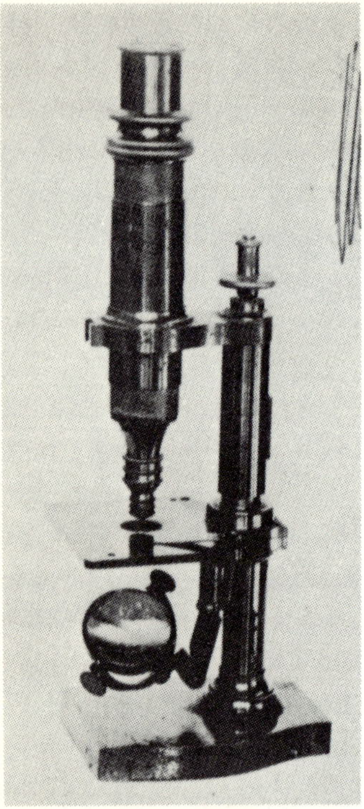

Microscope used by Pasteur most of his life. It lacks a mechanical stage, primary rack-and-pinion adjustment, objective turret, and a substage condenser, proving that it is the mind of the observer that counts rather than the apparatus

They were lactic acid ferments. The thought flashed through his mind that only the larger globules could make alcohol.

He could tell Monsieur Bigo this much. When the beet juice contained larger round globules, the fermentation would be healthy. When these globules became elongated, there was danger. When they became further elongated into little rods, the fermentation became lactic, sour and "sick." This did not, of course, solve M. Bigo's problem, but Pasteur's correct first guess put him on the road to a much greater discovery. But first he must get the proof.

No one would believe that ferments were alive. Liebig, the German chemist, would laugh at the idea. Apples rotted, meat spoiled, wine soured, and animals and people became sick, the way iron rusted or silver tarnished. Justus von Liebig would go on saying that all ferments were "nitrogenous matter," like the substance in milk, blood, or urine, which change when in contact with air.

To prove that each of the little beasts caused a specific kind of fermentation, Pasteur would have to separate them—grow them isolated from each other. He carefully laid his plans. First he had to find a way of clearing up the murky mess from the vats which made it almost impossible for him to see the myriads of rods. He would have to prepare some clear broth, and provide the little beasts with some special food to see if they would grow and multiply. He tried a sugar solution to which he added a bit of mixture scooped up from the "sick" vat. No, this wasn't the right fare; the little rods wouldn't grow. It must be that they needed a richer food.

Late in the night, long after Mme. Pasteur had put the children to bed, and had given up trying to tear her husband away from his bottles and smelly mixtures, he was struggling with various concoctions with which to tempt the microscopic specks. Finally, he boiled some dried yeast, strained it clear, and then added sugar and a bit of powdered chalk to keep his broth from being acid. To this mixture he added a tiny drop of the sick fermentation juice. He put the bottle in an incubating oven. Again he would have to wait—not hours but perhaps days.

The next day, weary with sleeplessness and worried over yet another failure to find a nutritious mixture for his elusive little rods, he went on with his business of lecturing to students, meeting with visiting businessmen, and carrying out his duties as Dean. The next evening he removed the bottle from the incubator. Something was happening. The mixture was clouding up, and bubbles were escaping. The following day there was a layer of foam, like the head in a stein of beer. He examined a drop as it spread on his slide under the lens. There they were, his tiny rods swarming by the million. "They are alive; they multiply!" he whispered, awestruck. Absentmindedly he answered his wife's call for dinner, but stayed at his microscope.

In the weeks that followed, he repeated the experiment, taking a drop from a flask that contained the little rods, and transferring it into another containing the clear yeast broth in which there were no rods. Each time, the rods grew by the billions. The amazing thing was that as they grew they produced lactic acid, the acid contained in sour milk. This is what made the beet juice sour and kept down its fermentation into alcohol. His hunch was right. "Keep the little rods out of the vats, and you will always get alcohol," he could advise the alcohol distiller. It was like keeping weeds out of a garden. But how? The answer might come later, but Pasteur was more concerned with his discovery.

Fermentation was caused by the little rod-shaped beasts. "Ferments" were alive! Let Liebig spout what he wants, but fermentation was caused by these bits of living things. Pasteur was beginning to see the answer to his own questions: "How explain the disintegration of a dead body or fallen plant? How account for the working of the vintage in the vat? Of dough left to rise and then souring? Of curdling milk? Of straw ripening on the dungheap? Of dead leaves and plants buried in the soil turning to humus?"

Liebig and his followers believed that fermentation was caused by contact with air and by albumin as a catalyzer. No one had ever seen living organisms in fermentations. But Pasteur's experiments with the little rods that produced the

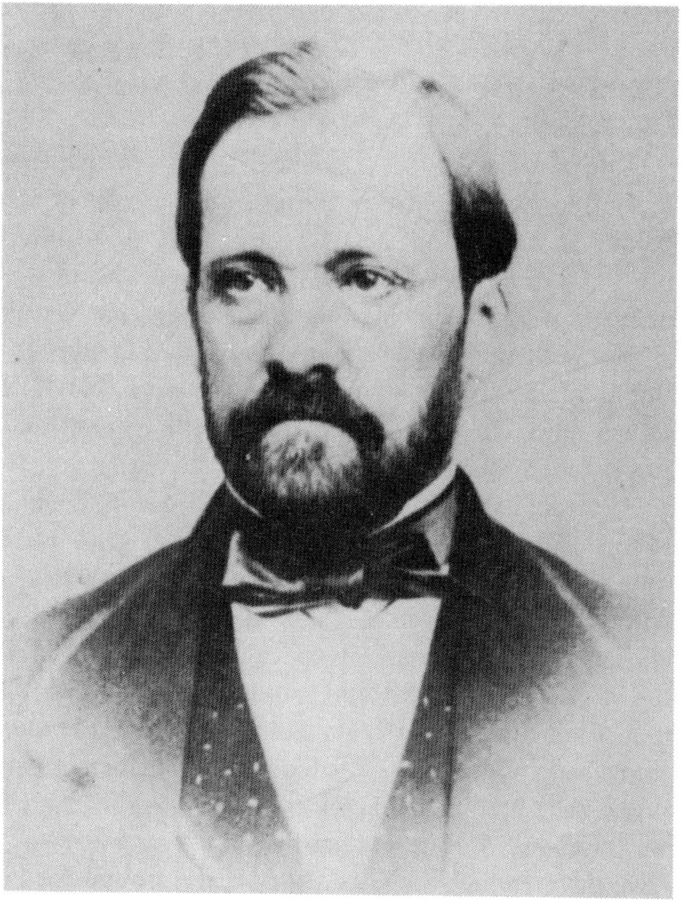

Rare portrait of Pasteur, made in 1857, the year of publication of his theory of the living cause of fermentation

acid in sour milk gave him the idea that these tiny beings must do other kinds of things, perhaps not always useful, and sometimes even dangerous. Only one way to find out—experiment! He was determined to find the proof that would fling the truth in the faces of his growing army of opponents who firmly believed that fermentation had nothing to do with living things. They were just as convinced that flies came spontaneously from dung, and fleas and lice "bred from dirt," and not from other flies, fleas, and lice.

One morning Pasteur announced to his wife that they were moving to Paris. He had been appointed Director of Scientific Studies at the Normal School, and despite their comfortable life at Lille, this was the chance he needed to find out what microbes were capable of, how they changed our very lives.

No well-equipped laboratory was awaiting him in Paris. But no matter. He would find a place to work. He did—a rat-ridden attic. Up the winding stairway he carried his microscope, flasks, tubes, and blast lamp.

He would show Liebig that yeasts do not need albumin to change sugar into alcohol. He would try to grow yeasts in a soup that contained no albumin. But yeasts were fussy eaters, and refused to work in one after another of his broths. Then one day he dropped some tartrate of ammonia in the broth, and the yeasts grew, budded, and multiplied luxuriantly. The ammonia salt disappeared as the yeasts flourished. He found the secret soup ingredients. Distilled water, ammonia salt, and sugar made up the fare on which the yeasts grew. No albumin was necessary. Liebig was dead wrong. Yeasts ferment sugar. Give them enough sugar and they make alcohol for months. It was these busy little globules which manufactured the millions of gallons of wine and converted barley sugar into beer in the giant brewery vats.

The first of his enemies—the Liebig disciples—bit the dust. Professor Dumas glowed with pride at his one-time pupil. The Academy of Sciences bestowed the Prize of Physiology, and the bearded Parisian professors proclaimed his genius. He accepted the praises naturally and confidently as he went about lecturing and reading defiant papers. To his father he reported Dumas' remarks: "... your audience this evening will applaud you as one of the most distinguished professors we possess." Indeed they did applaud his great researches with little beasts that turned butter rancid and others that made meat putrid.

Without living animalcules these things couldn't happen. He boiled his bottles of soups, milk, and urine, sealed the necks with heat, and set them on shelves. The contents of the flasks remained unspoiled for months, even years. When the bottles were opened there was no trace of microbes, and the air in the bottles retained all its oxygen. But the unheated, unprotected bottles swarmed with microbes, smelled putrid, and the oxygen in the flask had been used up. The organisms had used it up while burning the food Pasteur had furnished them. Here was proof that microbes caused souring, spoilage, and decay of food. In dozens of ways they worked *for* us in making wine, and *against* us in spoiling food.

But where did yeasts and other microscopic life come from? And why were they missing in the tubes he had heated? The glib answer others gave was Spontaneous Generation—another way of saying they sprang out of "natural" air. Pasteur had removed the *natural* air by heating his flasks, they argued. But Pasteur was convinced that by heating he had removed only the microbes.

He had to find a way to prove this beyond a doubt. M. Balard, one of his old professors at the Ecole Normale who followed the brilliant pupil's career, came to his aid. They put their heads together and found a way to keep out the germs but not the air. It was a simple trick—a gooseneck flask. With the heat of the blast lamp, he drew out the neck of the flask to a long curved tube, after half filling the flask with his mixture. He heated the flask to boiling, thus killing all the

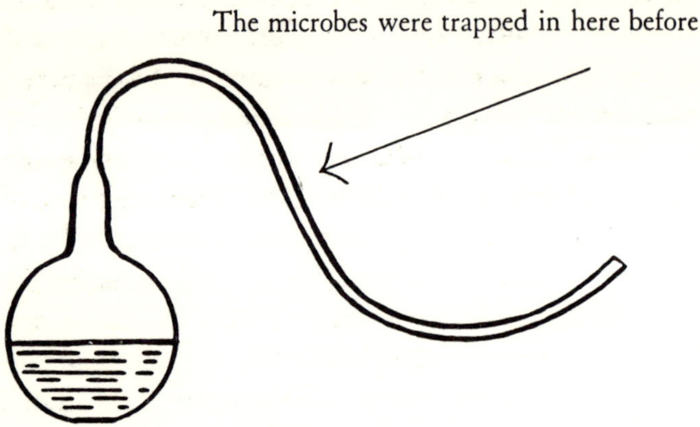

Pasteur's gooseneck flask

microbes in the broth, and driving the air out. When the flask cooled, fresh air could still come in through the open end of the gooseneck. But the microbes in the air could not get beyond the narrow, curved neck, so had no way of reaching the mixture. Weeks later, the bottles with the dry necks remained clear. In another set of flasks he let the soup run into the necks. In these, the microbes that were carried in with dusty air could swim into the belly of the flask and its contents became cloudy.

He proved that microbes could not come out of nothing. Once killed by heat, they could not grow again in the broth, unless there was access to dusty air that carried them in. They were everywhere, and Pasteur was sure that they must also cause disease. Before long he had the opportunity to prove it.

By the time Pasteur was 45 he had not only outwitted his scientific enemies, but had performed dramatic public experiments before the Academy of Sciences, been received by Emperor Napoleon III, and he had earned a reputation as an expert in diagnosing sick wines. If the winegrowers in Arbois didn't believe it, let them bring him bottles of wine that had gone bad with different diseases. Without tasting them, he would tell them if they were bitter, sour, or ropy. They tried to fool him, and give him a bottle of good wine among the rest. Sucking up a drop of each in turn and examining it under the microscope, he knew the good from the bad. What he saw under the microscope didn't fool him. More than that, he had a way to keep the wine healthy. If you heat the wine gently, way below the boiling point, the microbes that do harm to wine will be killed, he told them.

He earned the everlasting gratitude of the poor silkworm growers in southern France by finding that it was microscopic parasites that made their worms sick, lazy, and shrivelled, so that they wouldn't spin silk. He showed them how to examine the sick moths that emerged from the sick worms. The moths' bodies were full of tiny globules that made it necessary to discard the eggs they laid, for they would surely hatch into sick silkworms. Thus, Pasteur saved the French silk industry.

But always back of his mind was the persistent thought that microbes made not only wine, beer, and silkworms sick, but also people. Across the channel, in England, Sir Joseph Lister, the great surgeon, had made operations safe from infections that had previously killed eight out of ten patients even after successful surgery. In a letter to Pasteur, he acknowledged his debt to him. "Permit me to thank you cordially for having, by your brilliant researches, shown me the truth of the germ theory of putrefaction and for having given me the single principle which has made the antiseptic system a success." Inviting him to visit Edinburgh he went on, "I need hardly say

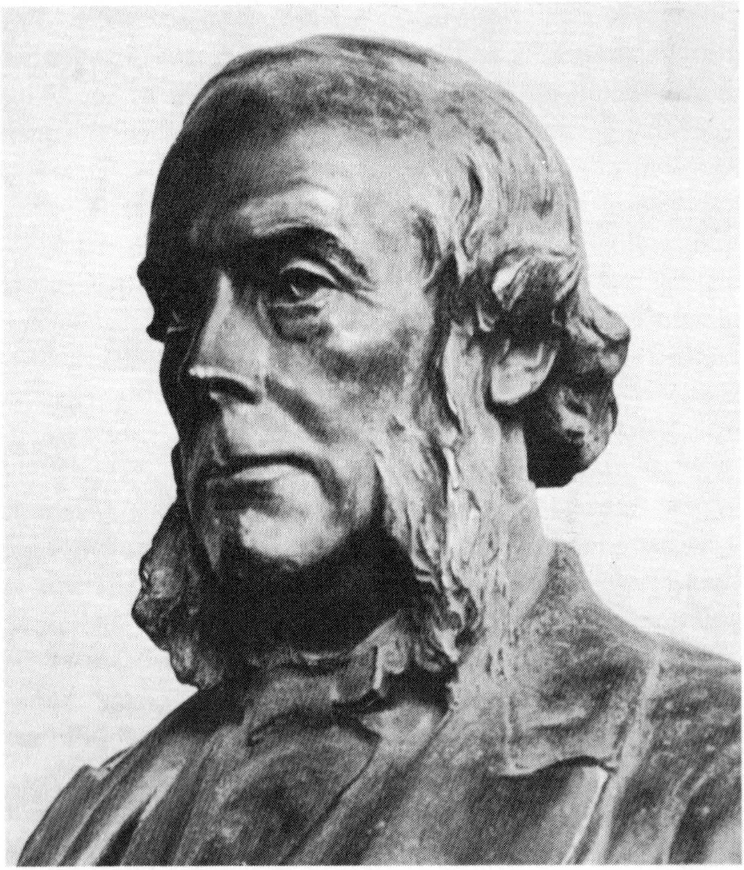

A sculptured bust of Joseph Lister, the "Father of Modern Surgery," in the National Gallery, London

that it would afford me the highest gratification to show you how greatly surgery is indebted to you."

By spraying the operating room, instruments, and even the operating field on the body with carbolic acid, the good surgeon was able to save hundreds of patients who would have died from infections. It was the miserable germs that caused the infections, and if you killed them, the wound had a chance to heal and the patient survive.

So far, Pasteur's ideas about germs in disease were little more than a hunch. By his penetrating studies on fermentation he had put microbes on the map. By 1870, the world was all agog with them. This hidden world of microbic life which he revealed with his microscope, and the billions of little energetic beasts he raised in his flasks, shared our air, water, soil, food, and everything else on our planet. Each was small and inconspicuous, but in groups and colonies these invisible neighbours put mould on bread and meat, raised dough, "aged" cheese, turned grapesugar into wine and wine into vinegar and perhaps also made healthy animals and people deathly sick. *"La vie c'est le germe et le germe c'est la vie,"* Pasteur said.

But while Pasteur insisted that microbes were murderers, responsible for epidemics and pestilences, the proof had yet to come. In the years that followed, he as well as others were to provide it.

4

VILLAGE DOCTOR ON THE ROAD TO FAME

Robert Koch (1843–1910)

ROBERT KOCH, a miner's son, stemmed from such humble folk that there is little known about his early life in Klausthal, northern Germany. He was one of thirteen children, and from a diary that his mother kept, we know that she educated them herself. With such a brood to look after, she had little time to keep young Robert out of all kinds of escapades—trapping and skinning cats, making outdoor meals on frogs and grasshoppers, and nearly bleeding to death once when he was caught on a hook in a tree he was climbing.

The Kochs lived the life of the poor, eating black bread and a little milk every day, with white bread reserved for Sundays. Sugar, coffee, and other delicacies were known only by reputation. Clothes were handed down, patches and all, from older to young. His father wanted Robert to be a shoemaker, but somehow things turned out differently.

Koch was born in 1843 at just about the time Pasteur came under the spell of M. Dumas' teachings at the Sorbonne. And when the French scientist was travelling the length and breadth of his country, saving the wine industry and studying the sickly silkworms that were too weak to spin cocoons, Koch was learning to be a doctor at the ancient University of Göttingen. He must have had some deep yearning to explore the world of science, to have found a way to study medicine. For after all, there was no rich father to send him to medical school.

Actually, Koch found little interest in memorizing the names of bones, muscles, and nerves which he conscientiously traced out in cadavers. His passion was mathematics and natural science. It was in the life sciences that he wanted to do his explorations, especially if it could take him to far-flung places. Perhaps learning to be a doctor would be a steppingstone to research. He dreamed of being a ship's surgeon—an occupation which would take him to strange places and also give him plenty of leisure to explore life.

He studied under the Berlin anatomist, Jacob Henle, who, even before Robert was born, had worked out the theory that infectious disease was carried by invisible forms of life. This idea was still scientific heresy, which is, perhaps, the reason it fired the imagination of such a thoughtful young man as Robert Koch.

But, somehow, fate didn't take him in that direction. When Koch graduated from Göttingen in 1866 he took his internship in an insane asylum in Hamburg. This was hardly a place in which to study the yet unknown world of microbes. The interne's job was to keep the raving and helpless patients from hurting themselves or one another. There was no hope of cures for the insane in those days. Confined to a madhouse, with all its demands on his time, the young doctor had little time or opportunity to keep in touch with the exciting discoveries Pasteur was making.

In 1870, when Prince Otto von Bismarck beat the war drums and sent a German army to invade France, young Robert Koch volunteered in the service of his country. The

Franco-Prussian war was over within a year, with the defeat of the French people by the professional Prussian army. Robert Koch, still dreaming of adventure in unexplored parts of the world, as he longingly watched the vessels departing from the Hamburg port, temporarily became resigned to the career of a country doctor. He was helped in his decision by Emmy Fraatz who agreed to marry him only if he gave up his foolish dreams of adventure far away from solid German soil.

Dr. Koch settled down as a district medical officer in the village of Bomst, not far from Breslau which was then Silesia. Here a conscientious doctor could build up a large, if not a rich practice. Besides, his duties as medical officer required that he travel in surrounding country. Emmy was satisfied with her

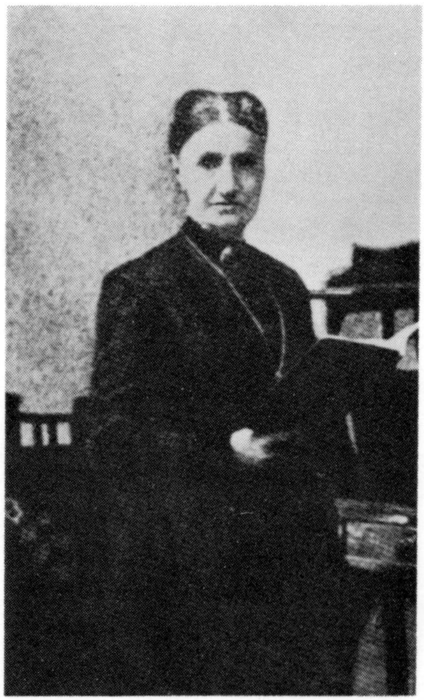

Robert Koch's wife, Emmy

marriage and proud of her husband who did what he could to comfort the sick and prolong the lives of the dying. But the doctor was restless.

There was nothing more discouraging to his searching spirit than having to make his calls on horseback, going from one farm house to another, prescribing the same old medicines or poultices. Isolated in a town with barely four thousand souls, he had almost no contact with the medical world that was beginning to buzz about the microbes scientists saw in their laboratories.

Casimir Davaine, a Frenchman, found little bodies he called "bacteridia," in sick animals. The sicker the animals, the more the little beasts that crowded their bloodstreams. Even a millionth of a drop of this diseased blood, when transferred into the blood of another animal, made it sick.

And C. J. Eberth in Germany proved that the substance that carried the disease could be separated from the blood.

In Scotland, Dr. Lister was saving the lives of mothers during childbirth by keeping the microbes away with his carbolic acid sprays.

In the medical colleges there was much talk about these killers, the microbes.

But Robert Koch had no way of hearing about such things in his country practice. When looking at his patients' tongues and counting their pulses seemed to him especially stupid, he would get off by himself and look at everything with an old magnifying glass.

When some child patient died of diphtheria after he had tried everything he knew, he would unburden his despair to simple Mrs. Koch who just looked puzzled at the fact that a man with all his medical training should feel so helpless. After all, who could do more? But then, when his twenty-eighth birthday came around, she bought him a microscope, in the same way that she would have bought a toy for a child. Could it even have entered her head that the gadget would start her husband off on his life adventures, more absorbing than a journey into the jungle?

At first it was hardly more than a fascinating hobby to put bits of tissue, pus, or urine on little plates of clean, shining glass, and peer for hours through his microscope as the beam of light was bent by the lens. Every moment he could take away from his doctoring, he devoted to his marvellous toy. Before long his chance came to use his instrument in disease.

Anthrax, a disease mainly of animals, was plaguing the sheep-raisers in Germany as it was in all Europe. It would go through a flock like smallpox in an army camp. No one could explain why a healthy sheep suddenly took sick, refused to eat, and the next day lay dead on its back with feet stiff as sticks, its blood turning black. Whatever the killer, it attacked sheep and cows, and even people who handled the animals. The victim could be the farmer who herded the animals, the wool sorter, or the dealer in hides. Sometimes they developed ugly boils; at other times they died from a severe disease of the lungs.

Koch decided he would look at a drop of blood from a dead sheep. He spread it on a glass slide and examined it under his microscope. Among the yellow discs—the blood cells—he saw much smaller short rods. Some seemed to be joined to form threads, others floated singly in the sticky fluid. Were these sticks alive? Were they the microbes Davaine had discovered in the blood of dead sheep? And did they cause anthrax? Davaine and Eberth got no further with their discovery of these little rods. Koch would study the problem himself. First he would find out whether the blood of healthy cattle contained the rods.

This was easy enough to do, even if the slaughterers thought the doctor was a bit queer for collecting the blood of freshly butchered animals. He took his little bottles home, and rushed to his precious microscope to look for the little rods. No, they were not to be seen in the blood of healthy animals. He would have to find out how they got into sick beasts, whether they grew there, in fact, whether they were even alive. His patients would have to wait. There was little he could do for them anyway. Only the little rods mattered.

He set up a makeshift laboratory behind a partition in his office. Here he would find out, experiment. No matter that in medical school he hadn't learned how, and that he would have to improvise some homemade apparatus. He could try to study these little rods in mice. He fed a little of the black blood from anthrax animals into the blood of his caged mice. The blood clotted and gummed up the needle. *"Ach, du Lieber,"* he would exclaim, but he didn't give up. He found it easier to make a cut in the tail of the mouse, and to introduce a bit of the poisoned blood with a clean splinter of wood soaked in it. Then he put the mouse back in its cage, washed his hands, and attended to a patient.

The next day he found that he had given the deadly disease to the mouse. There it lay, just like the dead lambs he had seen in pastures, stiff and blue. He fastened the dead mouse to a dissecting board, heated his knife, and slit the mouse open to examine its lungs, liver, and spleen. Overnight the spleen had crowded out the other organs. He cut into it with a heated knife, and picked up a bit of the thick black blood to put under his lens. Sure enough, the little threads he had dipped out of the dead sheep the day before had spread through the body of the mouse. There they had grown, multiplied by the millions and, finally, killed it. He transferred a bit of the black matter from the spleen of the dead mouse into the tail of another mouse, and the same thing happened. Each time he repeated the experiment, dozens of times and more, the little rods showed up in the last dead mouse. He was convinced he could spread the disease. The little threads must be alive, else how could several hundred on the tip of the wood splinter grow into billions in twenty-four hours?

How could he prove this? He couldn't look inside the mouse, and *see* them grow, as the animal became choked up with them. He would have to find a way to grow them outside the body. This meant finding the right kind of food for them, something that resembled the living body fluids. He decided the watery stuff that escaped from a cut ox-eye might be close enough. Then the little sticks would need warmth such as they found inside the mouse's body. He would have to make an incubator. His oil lamp would have to provide the heat under the drop containing the ox-eye liquid and the little beasts between the two bits of glass.

Then during the night he settled down to watch them multiply. Did they really grow? There seemed to be more of them, but he could also see intruders—other little beasts squirming and dancing between the rods. Somehow they had got in between the glass plates.

"How can I keep my little rods separate, away from the others?" he muttered to himself, and fumbled to find a way. When the idea finally came to him how to do this, he had discovered a method which is still in use today—the hanging-drop. On a thin piece of glass, the coverslip, which he had carefully heated to make sterile, he put a drop of his precious ox-eye juice; to this he added the tiniest bit of scraping from the spleen of a mouse that had died of anthrax. Then he took a thick slide with a scooped-out centre—a little bowl the size of a half-penny. All around this depression he spread some vaseline which would make the coverslip stick to the slide when he turned it over. When the coverslip and slide stuck together, he quickly inverted his apparatus, so that the drop with the culture "hung" down in the little well in the slide.

"This should keep out intruders from the culture, and enable me to study the little rods," he mused with eager anticipation.

He placed his slide onto the stage of his microscope and settled down to watch.

"Now, it should be possible to see if the little rods grow," he thought, as he tried to follow one little stick after another tangled in the mesh of spleen threads.

His eyes burned with fatigue, his spectacles clouded over with the moisture from his breath, and his straining neck muscles ached. The little beasts took their time as Koch gazed into the lens for a couple of hours, until things began to happen. The little rods began to stretch, lengthen, and divide—one into two, and two into four. He watched one and then another go through the same process of splitting, the numbers multiplying until they crowded out the bits of tissue on which they grew. So this was the way these little murderous bits of living thread choked the cells and blood channels of the animals they killed! Each by itself, too small to see—once it started off on its endless course of dividing and multiplying—could overpower a sheep a billion times as large! Because each little rod was alive and grew, it could kill. This was plain to Koch.

Where the little anthrax rods were concerned, the bespectacled doctor had endless patience. His practice lost all meaning, but the little rods held a fascination. He would see if he could make them continue to grow in pure culture. Each day he would transfer a bit of his hanging-drop containing some of the wiggling rods into fresh ox-eye juice, and watch them grow into millions and billions.

The last trace of the dead mouse's spleen had disappeared, and he had grown the microbes for eight generations, uncontaminated by any others. Only the little rods, descendants of the ones that had killed the mouse, were swimming in his hanging-drop.

"Would these bacilli still have the power to kill, if I injected them into a mouse or a sheep?" he asked himself. "Will they produce anthrax in a healthy animal?" This was the next question Dr. Koch had to answer.

He dipped a heated splinter of wood into the hanging-drop, and transferred the clinging bacilli into a slit in the skin of a healthy mouse. The next day he should know. Such answers had to be waited for patiently.

The next morning he slit open the mouse's belly and took a thin slice of the dead animal's spleen. In no time he was examining it under his lens.

"Here's the proof—the threads from the hanging-drop killed just as surely as the bacilli I first saw in the blood of the dead sheep."

After countless passages, each successive generation retained its deadly power to slay an animal as powerful as a cow! This tiny bacillus was the sure cause of anthrax!

Pasteur, with the vision of genius had looked into the future and had seen that microbes caused disease and destroyed their victims. In fact, he foresaw that "it is within the power of men to make parasitic maladies disappear from the face of the earth." But Koch was the first to prove that one kind of bacillus was the cause of one particular disease.

If Pasteur was the first to recognize the importance of his own discoveries, Koch seemed to be the last. Pasteur would burst with the news—shout from the housetops if necessary; Koch went on to dig deeper for answers, never even bothering to announce his discovery. How did anthrax enter the body? How did the bacilli go from the sick to the healthy? Why did they flourish in the body of a mouse but dry and perish on his slides?

Then the sheep herders and cattle men had other questions. How was it that in one pasture the animals remained well, and when driven to graze in fresh fields they fell from this dreadful plague? The herdsmen could only believe that their pastures were cursed. What else?

Koch was troubled. How, indeed, did these delicate threads survive the winter cold in the fields and mountains, and do their murderous job the following year? On his slide, they dried, faded, broke up, and the fragments injected into a mouse were harmless. In two days, they died on the slide, and in the fields they remained alive for months. There must be a reason!

Then one day, peering over a hanging-drop with anthrax bacilli which he had kept in his incubator for twenty-four hours, he expected to see a rich harvest of the beasts, because the incubator was the same temperature as the mouse's body.

"What could *this* be? Did some strange bugs invade my pure anthrax cultures?"

He had gotten to know his little rods like intimate friends, and what he saw seemed like intruders. They were oval glass-like beads ranged at intervals along the threads. When he studied them carefully he discovered that the bacilli had become transparent in spots, making the strands appear like beads on a string. He dried the drop and put the slide away. Sometime later he looked at it again only to see that the tiny beads were still there. He put a drop of the fresh ox-eye fluid on the dried material; before long the beads disappeared and he again saw the same rods he had come to know so well.

"How extraordinary. There must be a reason for this strange transformation—rods to beads, and beads back again to anthrax bacilli," he remarked with wonderment.

The thought struck him that the beads were *spores,* a form which these bacilli assumed under conditions which threatened their continued existence. Professor Ferdinand Cohn, a botanist at Breslau, who had made a name for himself by describing and classifying bacteria had also explained spores. Some bacteria turned into tough spores, Professor Cohn had written. This was perhaps the way anthrax bacilli resisted death, Koch guessed.

"Could this be the way these microbes kept themselves alive in the fields during the long winter months?" With the warmth of spring, did they become active, deadly bacilli once more? He would soon find out. He scooped out bits of spleen from mice that had died from anthrax, and stored the material on slides until the microbes had turned into spores. Then he put some of the fresh ox-eye juice on them and inserted a bit of the revived bacteria into the tail of a healthy mouse. Conditions were again favourable for their becoming active.

"This must be the answer. Spores never form in a live animal; only when it is dead, or when the blood is heated or suddenly chilled." Surely, this is what happens when a sheep, dead from anthrax, is left in a field. The bacilli change into spores. When the spores somehow get into healthy grazing sheep, they hatch into murderous rods, taking a new lease on life. It would explain how certain pastures became once more the "cursed fields" that the peasants dreaded.

It was time now for the modest doctor to make his discovery known to the scientific world, to show what he had learned about the life-history of the anthrax bacillus. The only way he could think of to do this was to send off a letter to Ferdinand Cohn, at the University of Breslau.

"Before, however, I bring this into the open, I respectfully appeal to you, esteemed Herr Professor, as the foremost authority on bacteria, to give me your judgment regarding this discovery . . . Should you, highly esteemed Herr Professor, be willing to grant my humble request, will you kindly appoint the time when I may come to Breslau?" Koch wrote.

Professor Cohn eagerly invited him to come to Breslau. In fact, Cohn was looking forward to the sensation Koch would create among the die-hard professors at the University—the backwoods common healer among the learned egg-heads. He sent out invitations to the most eminent of them. Let them come and raise their eyebrows.

Frau Koch, puzzled by her husband's queer preoccupation with scampering mice and dead animals, his smelly laboratory with its little glass dishes, wire hooks, and oil-stove incubator, was even more puzzled when she watched him pack these strange items into a suitcase. What baggage to take with him on a journey—a cage with white mice, glass slides holding deadly bugs, his precious microscope! He was off to the University of Breslau. It was 1876.

The learned professors had come prepared to look down their noses at the self-made scientist. What they saw and heard gave them an unexpected jolt. The quiet little man with gold-rimmed spectacles had no long-winded theories to expound. He was here simply to show them what he had done—the careful nursing of generations of little rods in pure culture from hanging-drop to hanging-drop. Deftly he transferred the microbes on wood slivers into the tails of mice; in myriads he recovered them from the spleens of dead mice; they could see for themselves the spores formed in the dried blood smears on the slides. For three days and nights he went on re-enacting his simple but painstaking experiments. Modestly he explained his gropings and revealed his astounding findings. What a show! It left the professors dumbfounded.

All had to acknowledge, though some did so grudgingly, that they had witnessed a tremendously important event in science. But the one who most warmly acknowledged Koch's contribution was Professor Julius Cohnheim, an eminent student of diseases. He jumped out of his seat and rushed to announce Koch's discovery to his students. "Go and see for yourselves what a man who taught himself the way to do research has discovered. Drop everything, and go see the marvellously simple and complete proof of his great discovery. I consider this the greatest discovery in the field of bacteriology and believe that Koch will again astonish and shame us with still further discoveries."

As the students filed into the hall they heard unassuming Dr. Koch drive home the simple fact: "Tissues from animals dead of anthrax, whether fresh, or putrid, or dried, or a year old, can only produce anthrax when they contain bacilli or the spores of bacilli . . . all doubt that these bacilli are the cause of anthrax must be laid aside."

From the results of his experiments logically flowed the method of preventing the spread of this dreadful disease. If all animals that died from anthrax were destroyed at once by burning, or by burial deep in the ground, where it is so cold that the bacilli cannot transform themselves into spores, there would be no way of spreading the disease to healthy cattle, he explained.

With one straightforward scientific fact Koch cleared away the superstitious rubbish about "cursed fields" and opened the way for a practical method of eradicating the spread of anthrax. The ways of medicine were bound to change—from guesswork to intelligent use of knowledge. Men could plainly see the enemy that brought disease. Having found a way to fight one, they should eventually be able to lick the rest.

What would happen to Dr. Koch? Having told the world of his discovery, would he go back to Wollstein and prescribe poultices for toothaches and powders for fevers? If Professors Cohn and Cohnheim had not interfered, Koch might have taken the next train home. But the two professors tried to persuade the government health authorities in Berlin that they should make it possible for Koch to continue tracking down disease germs. Germany should be proud of this man, they argued. Wasn't there a way for him to get freed of his country practice?

Their noble efforts brought Koch little more than what he had abandoned in Wollstein. The job as city physician in Breslau paid only a very small salary a year. The rest, it was expected, the newly famous doctor should collect in heavy fees from private patients. But if, thanks to his friends in Breslau University, his reputation as a brilliant discoverer travelled all the way to Paris, it brought no patients to his door. After a year or two of disappointment in Breslau, Robert Koch packed his belongings and took his wife back to Wollstein.

Nothing could keep him from his microscope and incubator and the absorbing world of nearly invisible living things. He found a way to stain them with dyes of different hues which distinguished one kind from another. Perhaps if he photographed these strange beings he could convince people that germs were a matter of life and death to them. So he bought a camera and attached it to his microscope. The pictures would tell the story. No one could then deny what so far he alone saw. Photographs would speak with a greater eloquence than words, at least than Koch's words. He was not a rabble-rouser like that Frenchman, Pasteur.

Two more years went by, and Dr. Koch was still watching, counting, and photographing his strange microbic world, when word came from Berlin that he had been appointed Extraordinary Associate of the Imperial Health Office.

His Breslau champions had helped to make Koch's dreams come true. In 1880 he moved to a well-equipped laboratory. No makeshift apparatus here. He had two assistants, the faithful Gaffky and Loeffler, at his side; there were no helpless patients to plague him, and no money worries to keep him from his work. This was a researcher's Paradise.

So convinced was Koch that each disease must be caused by its own specific germ that he believed the only way to track down any one killer was to grow it isolated from all others. Grow germs pure. But how? How keep out invaders that strayed into his tubes from the air, from the water in which he washed his glassware, from the food he furnished for his microbes?

While worrying about this problem he walked into his laboratory one morning and saw a slice of boiled potato on his work table. It was spotted with different coloured round specks like bits of spattered paint, each distinct from the other. He decided to have a look at a bit of each speck under his microscope. He heated the end of a fine wire, dipped it into a coloured mass on the potato, and then stirred the tip of it into a drop of water on his slide. To his amazement, when he examined the drop with his lens, it was swarming with bacilli—all of one kind. These must be germs that dropped onto the potato from the air, *and yet they were all of a kind*. He repeated the experiment with a bit of slime from another coloured speck, and found a different kind of microbe. Again each was like the one next to it, but distinct from those in another coloured speck. Here were the pure cultures he was looking for! Each coloured speck was a *colony* of a different species of bugs!

He called in his two assistants and explained to the astonished young men the meaning of his chance discovery.

"When germs from the air drop into a liquid broth they mingle and swim freely like fish in a pond. You can't separate the different kinds in a mixed culture. But if these same bugs fall on a solid surface, each sticks to the spot where it falls. Here it divides and grows into millions of the *same* kind. You see, on this potato, each type grew into a colony separate from every other colony."

It seemed so simple as to be unbelieveable. Was the master really right? The three got to work to test out his simple explanation. They mixed several kinds of germs in a flask of broth from which it would be impossible to fish each out separately. Then they dipped a wire into the flask and drew the tip of it across the cut flat surface of a boiled potato and waited for the bugs to grow. Where each kind stuck to the potato, a speck formed—a *visible colony*. When they examined a bit of each under the microscope, the germs in each colony were distinct. They had been grown *pure*. All of one kind in each colony!

Growing germs pure was only a matter of growing them on solid food! Koch then took some gelatin, the stuff from boiled bones, gristle, and tendons that makes jelly desserts jell. He dissolved gelatin in meat broth and boiled it until it was sterile. When it was cool, this solid, firm jelly made a nutritious

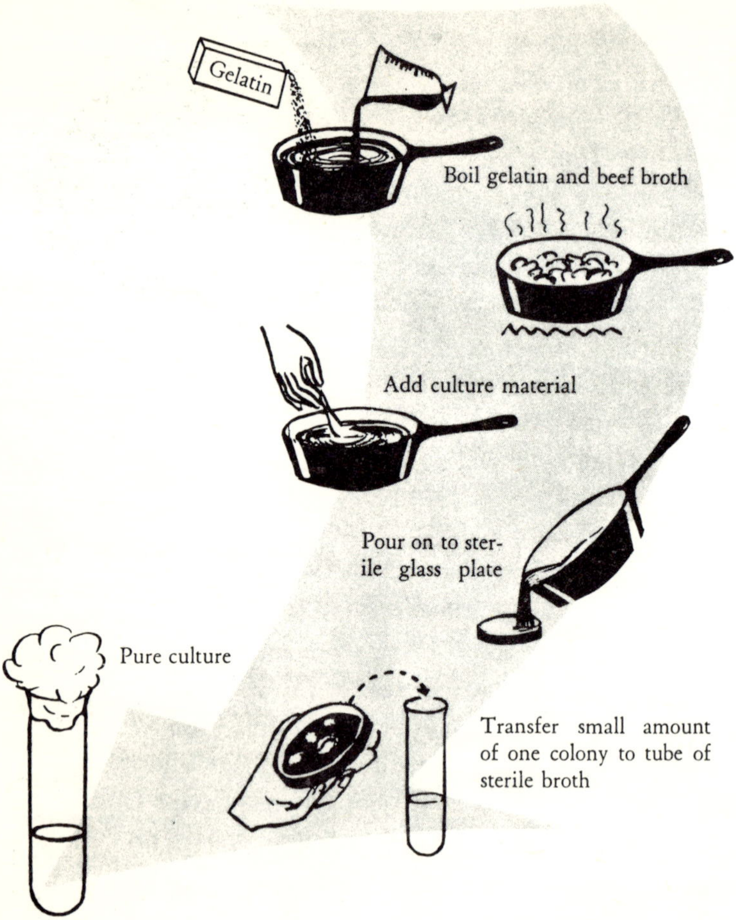
Gelatin
Boil gelatin and beef broth
Add culture material
Pour on to sterile glass plate
Pure culture
Transfer small amount of one colony to tube of sterile broth

Koch's method of isolating a pure culture

medium for his microbes. Then he added a bit of material from which he wanted to isolate a pure culture to the dissolved gelatin, and poured the mixture into a sterile dish. When the plate was cooled and the gelatin solidified, the suspended bacteria

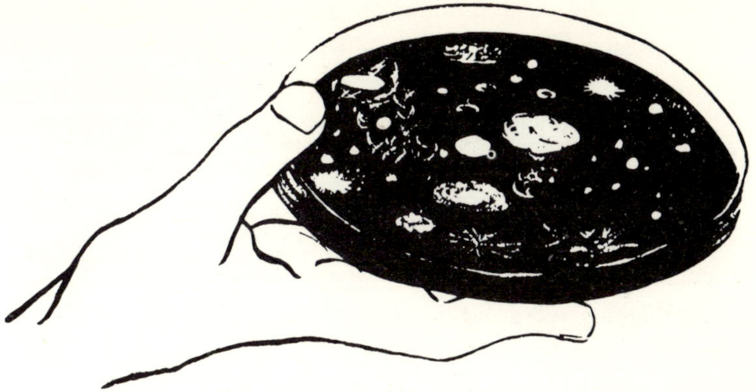

Colonies of bacteria on an agar plate

became fixed, each in its own spot on the gelatin plate. After a few days, each tiny cell had repeatedly divided until the millions together formed a visible speck, a pure colony on the gelatin plate. It was now possible to transfer a tiny amount of this colony into a tube of sterile broth, and grow the organism in pure culture in a liquid medium.

There was only one trouble with Koch's solid medium. When he incubated his bacteria at about 100 degrees Fahrenheit, the gelatin was no longer solid, so that the germs would not remain fixed in separate colonies. Then the wife of one of the laboratory workers who prepared the gelatin media had an idea. She recalled that her Dutch friends in Java thickened soups with agar which they obtained from plants called algae. When agar is dissolved in water it thickens into a jelly which remains solid even at incubator temperatures. Mrs. Hesse's idea—to use agar instead of gelatin—solved happily the problem of growing bacterial colonies luxuriantly and separating them at the temperature suitable for their growth.

Next, Koch decided to tackle one of the worst diseases man has ever known—tuberculosis. It was a pretty good guess that a microbe was the culprit, because rabbits inoculated with bits of sick lung tissue acquired the disease. Koch knew of Professor Cohnheim's experiment with tuberculosis which he induced in rabbits. The Breslau professor inserted a bit of diseased tissue into the cornea of a rabbit's eye. Through this transparent tissue he could watch the growth of tubercles as through a window. The tubercles were little diseased knots that spread in the rabbit's eye. Dr. Koch had a hunch that a germ must be lurking wherever this disease occurred, but the proof was not as easy as in anthrax, where the bugs swarmed in the blood and tissues of dying animals. To Koch, tuberculosis was an even greater challenge than anthrax.

First, he would have to get hold of some of the disease-producing stuff. The opportunity came when a healthy man suddenly developed a cough, a fever, night sweats, and pains in the chest. He had what people called "galloping consumption," because the tissues rapidly wasted away. Within a few days the patient died, and his lungs were full of tiny, grayish-yellow specks, the telltale tubercles. Koch obtained some tubercles from the dead man's tissues and crushed them with sterile knives. Then he injected some of this material into the eyes of rabbits and under the skin of guinea pigs. He would watch the disease develop in his caged animals. In the meantime, he examined dozens of slides on which he spread the crushed material from the tubercles of the dead man. But nothing showed up in his microscope. Koch wouldn't give up, so sure was he that the little beasts should be there. If only there were a way of making them come into view!

Then he remembered a young man he had met in Breslau —a student who was experimenting with dyes and tissues.

"Why not try staining the bugs with a dye that would make them stand out?" thought Koch.

He carefully spread the grains of a crushed tubercle on slides, and then soaked them in a blue dye for days. When the tissue had soaked up the stain, he put his slide under his microscope. Sure enough, there they were. Tangled among the sick lung cells were clumps of the thinnest little bacilli he had ever seen—tiny rods coloured blue. Compared with these the anthrax germs were giants, and these little rods were curved, not straight like the anthrax bugs. He could hardly believe that this was the tubercle bacillus!

He would be able to find out from his caged animals if these were really the killers. Weeks had now gone by and the once frisky rabbits were a sorry sight. Their shiny fur had lost its sleekness, the skin hung loosely on their bones, and their feverish bodies were wasting away. Before long they died.

With the skill he had developed over the years Koch pinned one of the little bodies on his dissecting board and cut it open with a heated knife. Inside he found the same gray tubercles he had first seen in the dead tuberculous man. Methodically, he repeated the procedure of crushing the tubercles, staining the smear on his slide and examining the specimen under his microscope. Again he saw the bent little sticks that he had separated from the sick man's lung.

This was it—the tubercle germ! He hurried into the next room to call Loeffler, who was searching for the diphtheria bacillus. It was as if he needed an on-the-spot witness to his discovery. Here was the proof before their eyes! From the bit of tubercle taken from the dead man, the germs had grown into billions and spread to the bones, joints, and even the brain of the rabbits and guinea pigs. The tubercle bacillus had eaten away at their tissues until the animals died.

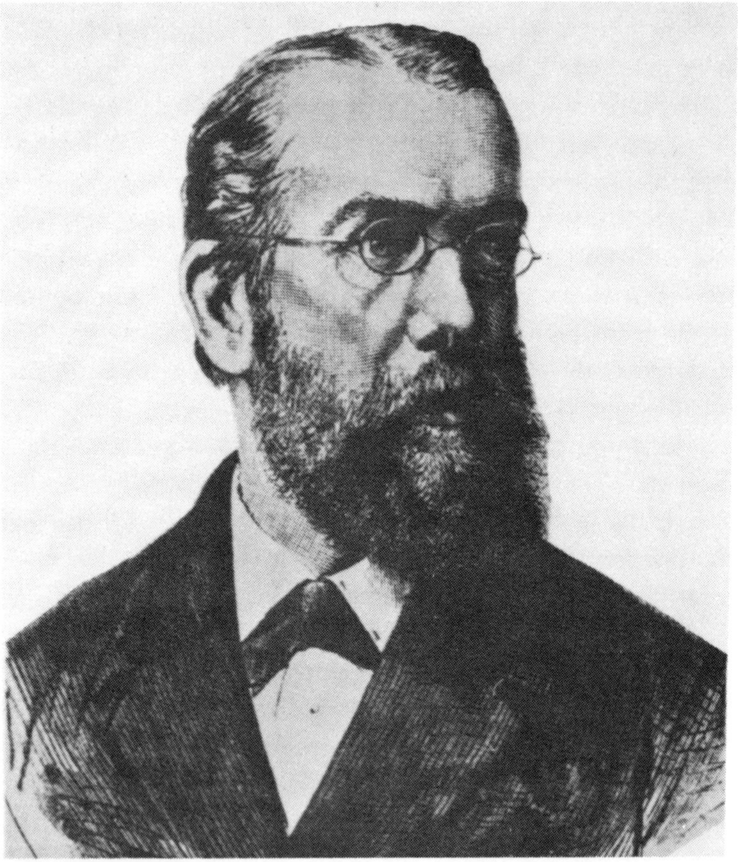

Dr. Robert Koch

From then on there followed a seemingly endless number of experiments in which Koch obtained more tubercles from persons who died from tuberculosis and injected the material into numberless animals—mice, rats, chickens, cats, and dogs. There was no let-up to this backbreaking and dangerous work. He could easily have contracted the disease himself. All that was needed was a slip of the syringe needle into his own hand, which would have carried the deadly germs into his blood. Time and again he would dip his hands into the strong bath of bichloride of mercury to avoid contamination.

Hundreds of times he found the curved thin little rods in the tissues of diseased animals, and never in healthy ones. Koch was convinced that he had found the cause of tuberculosis but he would have to do still more work to give complete proof to the most sceptical of critics.

With his usual thoroughness he worked out a set of rules for establishing final proof that a particular germ caused a certain disease.

Rule 1. Find the microbe present in diseased animals.

Rule 2. Isolate the microbe from these sick animals.

He had carried out rules 1 and 2. But that was not enough. He would have to go on to:

Rule 3. Grow the germ in pure culture and

Rule 4. Produce the original disease in healthy animals by inoculating them with the microbe.

With the tubercle bacillus, Rule 3 presented a stumbling block. He could not grow the bacillus in any of his beef broths, no matter what combinations he concocted. The bacilli just would not grow in his soups.

He puzzled and fretted over his failure, but stubbornly refused to give up, until suddenly he hit on an idea.

"It must be that these tubercle bugs will grow only in living tissue; the little devils are true parasites."

What could he prepare for them that would be closest to the living cells, or tissues? He would try blood. He collected quarts of blood from slaughter houses, allowed it to clot, and then siphoned off the clear, yellowish fluid that oozed out of the clot. This was blood serum which jelled into a soft, clear clot when allowed to stand. When he put the tubes on a slant he had a long flat solid surface of jelly on which to grow his germs. On this surface he streaked a bit of the tubercular tissue and put the tubes into the incubator.

It was a long wait before anything appeared on the jellied surface. The tubercle bacillus would have tested the patience of any other scientist, but not Koch. It took two full weeks before the glistening specks appeared. When he stained a bit of this material, scooped up on his heated platinum wire, he recognized the curved rods he was looking for. There was only one more step to the final test.

"I will slip a bit of this pure culture into the body of a healthy animal. If it develops the disease, then I will surely know that my bacilli are the cause of tuberculosis."

Again he repeated the injections into a still larger menagerie of every kind of animal he could collect, including those cold-blooded beasts—frogs, goldfish, eels, and turtles—that do not ever get the human form of the disease naturally. These did not succumb, but his mice, guinea pigs, rats, and monkeys did. He had followed his experiment to the last rule. This was the final proof!

In 1882, when Robert Koch announced his discovery of the tubercle bacillus, the scientific world was agog with the news. He was no longer the obscure village doctor, once a curiosity among professional scientists, but had joined the ranks of leading bacteriologists. In fact, the students who flocked from all of Europe, America, and Japan to learn from the wizard of Berlin, called him the Father of Bacteriology. The German Government sent him to Egypt to study another human scourge.

While Koch is in search of other disease germs, our story takes us back to France, where the fight against anthrax had its finish.

5

SHOTS THAT HEAL

Pasteur Continues

ONE WOULD have thought that Koch's crystal-clear and logical experiments should have demonstrated once and for all that the little rods caused anthrax; that the spores were like seeds which remain inactive until they fall on soil where they can germinate. But there were many doubters and much confusion. Some argued that the real cause was not the germ but some contagious matter, a mysterious "virus" which since the end of the sixteenth century meant a slimy poison. This virus was not visible in the blood, they said. Others claimed that the germ was merely a way of transferring the virus. Meanwhile, in the French sheep-growing provinces twenty out of every hundred in a sheep flock died, losses that cost millions of francs each year. Pasteur decided that before the problem could be solved, the idea that germs caused disease would once and for all have to be settled.

In 1878, he wrote to his old Arbois school fellow, Jules Vercel:

"I am extremely busy; at no epoch of my scientific life have I worked so hard or been so much interested in the results of my researches, which will, I hope, throw a new and a great light on certain very important branches of medicine and surgery."

Unlike Koch, who ploddingly worked out every step of an experiment, trying to anticipate all possible doubts and criticism, Pasteur took on his adversaries wherever he met them. He would first dispose of this notion that there was an evasive virus apart from the bacilli which everyone admitted seeing.

He prepared a culture fluid, to which he added a single drop of blood taken from an infected animal. From this fluid, which soon was teeming with anthrax bacilli, he took another drop which he put into a fresh supply of culture medium. Again and again he transferred a drop into yet another culture, forty and more times. Surely the so-called virus must have disappeared with all these successive dilutions. Yet injection of the last transfer was found to be fatal to rabbits and guinea pigs. Here was the evidence that the virulence could not have come simply from some elusive product in the first drop of blood. The strength of the fortieth and even hundredth transfer could be due only to the presence of live bacilli which continued to develop in each successive medium.

He provided yet more proof that germs were the sole cause of disease. He cooled the flask containing a culture of anthrax bacilli, to make the germs sink to the bottom, leaving the upper part of the liquid sterile. When he inoculated animals with the liquid alone, he found it powerless. But a sample from the bottom of the vessels, where the bacilli had collected, proved fatal to the injected animals.

Again there were objections. To be sure the animals died, but after awhile there was no trace of the bacillus in their blood. So he boarded the next train to Chartres to meet his opponents on the spot where infected animals had died. There he examined the blood of animals that had just expired. Their blood swarmed with anthrax bacilli, while other carcasses, many hours after death, revealed none. Here he made an important discovery. A new type of organism, which usually lives in the intestine, penetrated into the blood after death. These were capable of developing without air and grew into vast numbers. When such blood, freed of anthrax bacilli that got their oxygen from the living tissues, was injected into animals, it killed them, but not from anthrax.

Another argument cropped up. One experimenter collected diseased blood and destroyed all the bacilli with compressed oxygen. Yet animals inoculated with this seemingly disease-free blood developed anthrax. It must be that something other than bacilli was the cause. Pasteur had an answer for him as well.

He invited him to his laboratory where he showed him that although compressed oxygen killed the bacilli, it had no effect on the development of spores. Q.E.D. This time his opponent admitted his error. But there were many more who did not, which kept Pasteur's fertile mind one mental hop ahead of the doubters and critics.

One of Pasteur's oft-repeated sayings was that chance and accident proved useful only for the mind that was prepared for them. One such chance observation was to lead Pasteur to one of his greatest discoveries.

Koch had his devoted Gaffky and Loeffler, and Pasteur his Chamberland and Roux, two brilliant young physicians. Wrote Roux: "Chamberland and I settled here. . . . Pasteur came every week to superintend and examine our investigations. We have many memories of that campaign against anthrax in the

Chartrian district. In the early morning we visited the sheepfolds scattered over the wide plateau of the Beauce, shining in the glory of the August sun; then we carried out autopsies in the knacker's* yard or on the farms. In the afternoons we recorded our experiments in the notebook, wrote to Pasteur, and planned new researches."

Pasteur depended on these young physicians. For one thing, since he had been trained as a chemist, he needed their skills and knowledge of medicine to collect specimens from hospital patients, to do post-mortems, and even to jab needles into guinea pigs and rabbits. The business of dissection was especially distasteful to him, and he loathed hospitals with their sickly smells especially when he was engaged in the study of childbirth fever, and had to frequent the unsanitary maternity wards.

Working with a master as versatile as Pasteur made life exciting for the bright doctors. Before long they were investigating a new malady—chicken cholera, a highly contagious disease of fowl. Quite suddenly the chickens would become sluggish in their movements, and sit quietly with their drooping heads sunk into their ruffled feathers. About nine-tenths of a brood would drop off in an epidemic, but those who survived were usually immune to another attack. In the midst of the battle against anthrax, Pasteur turned his attention to chicken cholera.

A veterinary in Turin had described the organism, and Pasteur began to cultivate it pure in a broth made of chicken gristle. When he inoculated hens with his thriving cultures, they invariably became ill, while the same injection into a guinea pig caused only a local abscess, but no other effects of

---

*One who buys worn-out horses for their hides and hoofs.

illness. A chicken put into the same cage with the guinea pig contracted the disease from the otherwise normal rodent and promptly died. Perhaps a less observing experimenter would have decided in favour of the spontaneous origin of the disease in the fowl, but not Pasteur. He knew that the tiny guinea pig abscess carried the virulent organisms.

Day after day, and week after week, Roux and Chamberland nursed the tiny poisonous bugs, transferring a drop from one flask to another with fresh broth, breeding billions of them. Each culture was as potent as the one they isolated from the first sick hen.

The business of culture transferring went on for months, and the flasks accumulated, some of them containing cholera germs several weeks old. It was time to get rid of the older ones, when Pasteur instructed Roux to try one of them on a few chickens. As usual the birds became drowsy, and dropped off in a corner of the cage looking sick. By next morning they should have been dead, but strangely enough they perked up as if nothing had happened. What could be the meaning of this? Out of every dozen inoculated, twelve chickens had always before been stretched out dead the next day, but not this time.

Then it seems that vacation time rolled around, Pasteur and his assistants went away, and the laboratory was temporarily left in the hands of the caretaker.

On his return, Pasteur asked that some healthy chickens be made ready for inoculation. He was reminded that most of the chickens had had the old cultures, and no new supply of healthy ones had been obtained.

"Oh, yes, of course, but let's try shooting some fresh culture into them, and also some of the same in the few healthy ones," Pasteur decided.

In the morning when Pasteur appeared in the animal room, there were the few "healthy" chickens stretched out stiff, and the ones that had recovered from the effect of the old cultures pecking away at their food as normal chickens should. Pasteur could hardly contain himself until his assistants arrived to see what he saw. To his annoyance Roux and Chamberland stood there wondering at their master's agitation.

To Pasteur the meaning was all too clear. "It's simple. Reduce the strength of the culture, just enough to make the animal a little sick. Then he will recover, and he will be able to take another virulent dose without getting the disease."

To the astounded young men he went on explaining his discovery—greater than Jenner's—because Jenner knew nothing about germs. If a way can be found to weaken microbes—by aging, taming, reducing their strength with chemicals—"we can turn them against themselves," he shouted. A vaccine can be made to immunize against disease. What a way to save lives!

"We will try it with anthrax," said Pasteur.

The drive to make vaccine was on. Pasteur's laboratory was buzzing with activity. Night and day the men worked to produce different potencies of the vaccine: the one that killed mice would just make guinea pigs sick; the one that poisoned a guinea pig would be too weak to do harm to a rabbit. When they had a row of flasks with anthrax cultures weakened to varying degrees by exposure to temperatures of $43^{\circ}C$, they would shoot first the weakest into a sheep, making it just a bit sick; when it recovered, it received a stronger dose from which it also recovered. In the end it could withstand what would have been a murderous dose for a cow.

Pasteur lost no time in announcing to the Academy of Sciences that he could prevent anthrax in cattle and horses. But more, he had no doubt that vaccines could be produced for any disease. His unshakeable confidence very nearly frightened his listeners. What made him so sure? Worse than that, he antagonized the veterinarians. What was all this bluster about saving everything that crawls and leaps? Did he think he was God?

Then the Agricultural Society of Melun decided they would challenge Pasteur to a public demonstration. Let Pasteur show what he could do. If by some chance he was right, they had nothing to lose but the money they put up to buy the necessary cattle. If he failed, then they would hear no more of his bragging. Pasteur jumped at the idea. Why not?

The public experiment was set to take place in May and June of 1881 at the farm of Pouilly le Fort, near Melun. Pasteur's friends feared for him, one of them gently warning: "You remember what was said of Napoleon: that he liked hazardous games with a touch of grandeur and audacity. It was neck or nothing with him, and you are bound for the same course."

But Pasteur was unshaken. "What was successful in the laboratory on fourteen sheep will be just as successful at Melun on fifty."

Even Roux and Chamberland, who were recalled from a much needed rest, were nervous and worried that perhaps their master was risking his reputation as a scientist. The Veterinary Press carried a lead article about the discovery that was about to be tested—a vaccine against the most dreaded of animal diseases, one that even hit men.

On May 5th a vast crowd of doctors, veterinarians, agriculturalists, and reporters assembled in the field at Pouilly le Fort. There were two camps: Pasteur's supporters tense with fear of failure, and his vicious critics delighting in anticipation of his downfall. Only Pasteur, Roux, Chamberland, and Thuillier, the youngest assistant, went about their business with the confidence of men who know their parts.

Fifty sheep were divided into two flocks. Twenty-five were treated with five drops of a weakened (attenuated), culture, and the other twenty-five were set aside as the controls. One ox and five cows also were injected with the vaccine. While the dumb beasts were returned to their sheds, Pasteur entered one of the large rooms at the farm to address a crowd of interested listeners. As if he were lecturing to a class of students, he calmly explained his experiments that had culminated with his discovery of the anthrax vaccine.

Unperturbed by questions and objections from the crowd, he defended neither his method nor his reputation. He was there to give the world the benefit of laboratory findings, to save the sheep and cattle raisers of France from utter ruin. This was not an argument between him and his opponents; he was defending Truth against Prejudice.

The second part of the experiment took place on May 17th. A second inoculation with a vaccine that retained more of its original potency was given to the same animals as before.

The final test came two weeks later. Again, there was a huge gathering, most of whom came to see the Big Show that they were sure would end in a grand fiasco for the chief actor. Prior to the enactment of the final scene, two of the unvaccinated and two vaccinated sheep had been given a strong dose of deadly anthrax. By the time the spectators, including a number of dignitaries, had arrived, the two vaccinated sheep were grazing unconcernedly, while the two unvaccinated ones lay dead.

Then the remaining forty-six sheep and all the cattle, both

the vaccinated and the controls, were brought into the field, and each received the fatal dose of virulent anthrax bacilli from the syringe in Roux's skilful hand.

During the next two days and nights there was a hush in the laboratory back in Paris. Pasteur himself spent a sleepless night, and, as Roux said, "His faith staggered for a time, as if the experimental method could betray him." And Mme. Pasteur, writing to her daughter, told of their fear of a possible last-minute disaster: "Your father would not let his mind be distracted from his anxiety."

But on the appointed day when the results were to be in, and Pasteur and his assistants entered the farmyard, a murmur of applause burst into a loud acclamation from the immense crowd. Twenty-two of the twenty-four unvaccinated sheep lay dead, and two were breathing their last. All the vaccinated sheep were in perfect health. The same clear-cut result was plain to see among the cattle.

One of the previously sceptical veterinarians stepped up to Pasteur to acknowledge: "I am a converted and repentant sinner," to which the scientist replied: "Permit me to quote you the words of the Gospel: 'Joy shall be in heaven over one sinner that repenteth more than over ninety and nine just persons which need no repentance.' "

Pasteur's method of attenuating deadly germs, as if forcing them to protect their attackers, had triumphed. As the victor was escorted to the train, the admiring shouts told of the conversion from doubt to certainty, from ignorance and helplessness to knowledge and power.

The most confirmed opponents now became the most enthusiastic supporters. Through the length and breadth of France, hundreds of thousands of sheep and cattle were being vaccinated.

When the Government bestowed upon Pasteur the Grand Cross of the Legion of Honour for service to his country, he laid down as the condition of acceptance that Roux and Chamberland should receive the Cross or the Red Ribbon of the Order.

To Pasteur, the world owes the method of protecting animals and men against a deadly disease, and to Koch the proof of the anthrax bacillus as the sole source of the infection.

Anthrax was conquered and Pasteur was impatient to tackle yet another enemy—the germ of rabies, the mad dog disease. He knew he could leave to his faithful assistants the business of cooking up the anthrax vaccine by the gallon. And they did their job skilfully and tirelessly. In answer to the thousands of calls for vaccine, Roux, Chamberland, and Thuillier took turns at making the lifesaving stuff and hurrying off to farms, miles away from Paris, to inoculate sheep by the hundreds.

With the crude apparatus in Pasteur's little laboratory, and the insane rush to make all of France's sheep safe from anthrax, something was bound to go wrong. Complaints began coming in of sheep dying, not as before—from anthrax picked up in the field—but from the vaccine which should have made them immune. Evil tongues were wagging once more; the vaccine didn't work, they insinuated. Pasteur was disheartened over the losses, but not shaken. With the confidence of a gambler who is certain that his luck is only temporarily changed, he went on to proclaim to the world that it must put its hope in the principle of weakening microbes.

But Robert Koch, that infinitely careful and exacting experimenter, sat down and wrote a cool, piercingly logical report of his tests with Pasteur's vaccine. He found, in sampling the stuff, that the weakest wouldn't kill mice, and what should have killed only guinea pigs sometimes killed sheep. What made M. Pasteur think he had a pure vaccine? Why it swarmed with all kinds of bugs just as stagnant water did! The vaccine was contaminated or had lost its strength or, even worse, the bacilli had not been weakened.

Coming from Koch, known the world over for his meticulous accuracy, it was like a challenge to a duel, which Pasteur was ready to take up. Who was Koch anyway? The German had been hardly out of his knee breeches when Pasteur had prepared pure cultures, the volatile Frenchman raged.

There was right and wrong on both sides. Pasteur's vaccine had become contaminated and weakened, and Koch discovered this as the reason for the accidental deaths. Pasteur resented the harsh criticism by the man he considered his rival. On Koch's part the criticism was justified; but in pointing out the error, he perhaps allowed his personal feelings to enter the scientific argument. Besides, he gave ammunition to Pasteur's critics in France.

But Pasteur had also his seconds. French patriots, feeling their nationalistic pride hurt, rose to defend their country's hero. As if to fling the insult into the face of the German, the proud old men of the French Academy elected Pasteur to membership, according him the greatest honour a Frenchman can receive.

The inglorious incident over, Pasteur went on to perhaps his greatest achievement.

Monsieur Bourrel, an old army veterinary surgeon, who had been trying to find a cure for hydrophobia, or rabies, brought two mad dogs to Pasteur. Perhaps the great scientist would be more successful than he had been. Of course, Pasteur

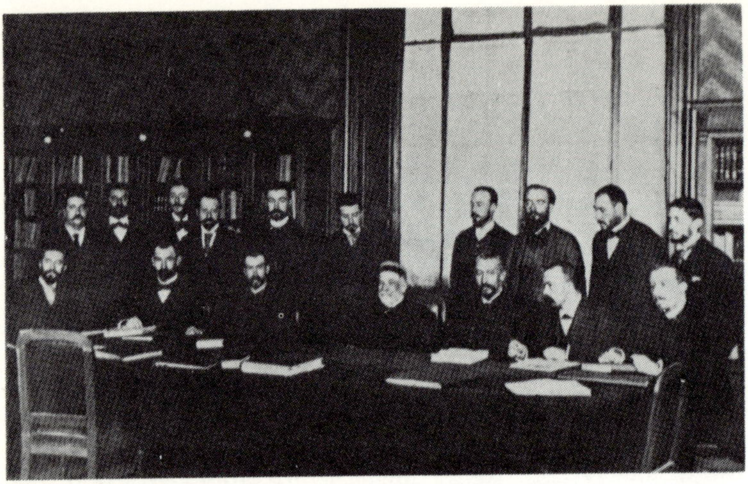

The last presidium attended by Louis Pasteur at the Academy of Medicine. At his left, Dr. Emile Roux

was immediately interested. The dogs' symptoms were unmistakeable: the half-opened, paralyzed jaws, froth-covered tongues, bloodshot eyes full of anguish. Furiously the beasts snatched at anything held out to them, and their despairing howls pierced the air.

Shortly afterwards Pasteur was informed of a five-year-old child who had been bitten on the face a month before, and had just been admitted to a nearby hospital. Restless, shuddering at the least breath of air, unable to swallow, yet suffering terrible thirst, the patient soon showed convulsive movements, then fits of rage, and died a day later. Pasteur gathered some of the saliva and mucus that filled the mouth of the choked child and took it to the laboratory to inoculate rabbits. The rabbits died within thirty-six hours, and so did other rabbits inoculated with saliva taken from the dead ones.

But Pasteur had reason to believe that these deaths were not necessarily due to rabies. The saliva contained an organism which he had found also in children who died from other causes; he found it even in healthy adults. Inoculation with saliva was also uncertain; sometimes it didn't produce the disease at all, and often it took weeks and months to develop. "We must try other experiments," Pasteur told Roux.

As he continued with the work he became more convinced that the rabies germ must grow in the nervous system. The anguish and fury, the change in the howl, the difficulty in swallowing, and finally the paralysis all pointed to the nervous system as the place where the microbe becomes lodged. "That is where we must look for it," he insisted. When he obtained some of the brain matter from a dog that died from rabies, and shot a little of this under the skin of normal animals, he was more successful in producing the disease.

"The seat of the rabic virus," Pasteur wrote, "is therefore not in the saliva only; the brain contains it in a degree of virulence at least equal to that of the saliva." But even then not all animals got the disease, and it took a long time to develop in others. "The incubation period must somehow be shortened; if only we could shoot it right into the brain." But how?

This is where Dr. Roux, the physician, could supply a method which Pasteur, the chemist, might not have thought of or would have been loathe to use. They drilled a little hole in the head of a chloroformed dog and injected a bit of the virulent matter right into the brain. The reasoning was clear: if it is in the nervous system where the disease ends up, it should develop more surely and quicker by this method. The animal that recovered from this operation almost immediately seemed no different from any other, until fourteen days later it began to tear its bed, showed delirious hallucinations, gave telltale howls, and finally came paralysis and death.

After several such experiments, Pasteur was able to say that the first step—producing the disease in animals—was accomplished. But the next step—isolating and growing the organism in pure culture in broth—eluded him. The reason was that he did not find the microbe. He was sure that it existed, but perhaps it was too small to see.

"Since this unknown being is living," Pasteur thought, "we must cultivate it; failing an artificial medium, let us try the brain of living rabbits."

Rabbit after rabbit was inoculated through a trephined hole in the head, with the material taken from the brain of the one that had just died. After one hundred such successive inoculations, the incubation period was reduced to seven days, and the virulence was greater than that of the virus in dogs that had become rabid through a bite.

Pasteur was able to control the strength of the virus, and to predict the time when death would occur in an inoculated animal. Now, the next step was to try to weaken the virus. If the virus could be attenuated, perhaps dogs could be made immune to rabies.

A fragment of the brain of a rabbit dead from rabies was suspended by a thread and placed in a sterile vial, in which the air was kept dry. After fourteen days, as this bit of tissue gradually dried, its virulence was gone. This inactive material was then injected under the skin of a normal dog. The next day he was given a similar dose of material that had been dried for thirteen days. Thus, by injecting daily gradually increasing strengths of the material containing the virus, the dog received on the fourteenth day the virus taken from a rabbit that had died on the same day.

Were the dogs now immune? It would be easy to find out. If the dog was placed in a cage with a mad dog, he would be bitten, or some of the rabies-producing material could be placed directly into his skull. Whichever way they used to test its immunity the animal resisted the disease.

Almost four years after the first lassoed mad dog was brought to the laboratory, Pasteur was ready to say that he had a dog immune to rabies. But, not wishing to repeat his experience with anthrax, he asked that a Commission be appointed to verify his results. In the spring of 1884, the Minister of Public Education arranged for a Commission of qualified men to repeat Pasteur's experiment.

The Commission met and elected a chairman who began his report: "M. Pasteur tells us that, considering the nature of the rabic virus used, the rabbits and the two new dogs will develop rabies within twelve or fifteen days, and that the two refractory dogs will not develop it at all, however long they may be detained under observation."

On the same day, Mme. Pasteur wrote to her children. "Nothing is settled as to commencing experiments. Your father is absorbed in his thoughts, talks little, sleeps little, rises at dawn, and, in one word, continues the life I began with him this day thirty-five years ago."

Through the next month, the experiments went on. Dozens of control dogs were given the test by being bitten by a rabid dog, while the two dogs that Pasteur said were immune underwent all ways to determine whether they were really vaccinated: bites, injections into the veins, and trephining.

By the beginning of August, the Commission's report went to the Minister of Public Instruction. "We submit to you today this report on the first series of experiments that we have just witnessed, in order that M. Pasteur may refer to it in the paper which he proposes to read at the Copenhagen International Scientific Congress on these magnificent results, which devolve so much credit on French Science and which give it a fresh claim to the world's gratitude."

Pasteur went on to Copenhagen where he was received with special honour by the King and Queen of Denmark and of Greece. Pasteur rose to thank the President of the Congress: "In the name of France. . . . By our presence in this Congress we affirm the neutrality of Science. . . . Science is of no country. . . . But if Science has no country, the scientist must keep in mind all that may work towards the glory of his country. In every great scientist will be found a great patriot. . . . Humanity then profits by those labours coming from various directions. . . ."

To wipe out rabies, Pasteur would have been ready to vaccinate every dog in France. But there were 100,000 dogs in Paris alone, two and a half million in the country. Each would have to receive several inoculations. Imagine the cost of caring for these dogs and the people it would require to carry out this colossal task. And where would one find enough rabbits in which to make the vaccines?

Such a project seemed altogether impractical. And then he thought of another way. If human beings could be made immune after they were bitten . . .

Writing to the Minister of Brazil, Pasteur said: "What I want to do is to obtain prophylaxis of rabies *after* bites. Until now I have not dared to attempt anything on men, in spite of my own confidence in the result of numerous opportunities afforded to me since my last reading at the Academy of Sciences. I fear too much that a failure might compromise the future, and I want first to accumulate successful cases on animals. Things in that direction are going very well indeed. . . ."

Another year went by. All kinds of difficulties arose in the

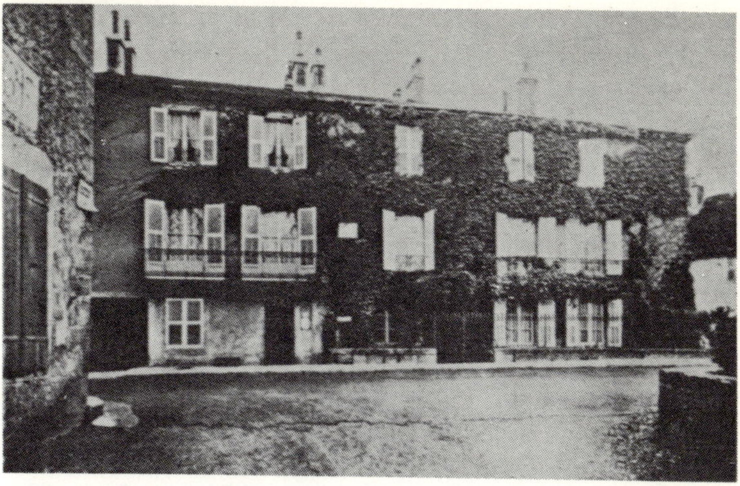

Pasteur's home at Arbois. Note plaque just left of centre

building of a kennel for his continued experiments. People in the neighbourhood chosen for this purpose raised a clamour concerning the danger to their children; imagine having rabid dogs so close to their homes, they protested. A place was finally located at Villeneuve L'Etang to house sixty dogs, fifty of which had been made immune.

Pasteur wrote to his old friend Jules Vercel that he would not be able to go to Arbois for Easter, because he was busy settling his dogs. "I have not yet dared to treat human beings after bites from rabid dogs; but the time is not far off, and I am much inclined to being myself inoculated with rabies, and then arresting the consequences; for I am beginning to feel very sure of my results."

Then one day Joseph Meister, a little Alsatian boy who had been bitten by a mad dog, was brought by his mother to Pasteur's laboratory. On his way to school he had been attacked by the dog which inflicted fourteen wounds on him. Pasteur was torn between trying preventive treatment on the child who would surely contract the disease, and the possible risk of failure. He consulted a member of the Rabies Commission, who felt that Pasteur's results were sufficiently conclusive for him to take the step. He ruled that it was actually Pasteur's duty to inoculate the boy, for this was the one chance of snatching him from sure death.

They began the inoculation with the fourteen-day-old virus which had already lost its virulence. The others followed in succession.

"All is going well," Pasteur wrote to his son-in-law five days later. "The child sleeps well, has a good appetite, and the inoculated matter is absorbed into the system from one day to another without leaving a trace. . . . If the lad keeps well through the following three weeks, I think the experiment will be safe to succeed."

In the meantime, as the inoculations were becoming more virulent, Pasteur was losing sleep from his anxiety over the outcome. "My dear children," wrote Mme. Pasteur, "your father has had another bad night; he is dreading the last inoculations on the child. And yet there can be no drawing back now!"

Thirty-one days after the child had been bitten he was still well and happy as he had been on his own farm. In the autumn of that year, three months after little Joseph Meister had been bitten, Pasteur reported his results to the Academy of Sciences. It was 1885, five years after Pasteur had begun the work on rabies. "From this day, humanity is armed with a means of fighting the fatal disease of hydrophobia and of preventing its onset. It is to M. Pasteur that we owe this, and we could not feel too much admiration or too much gratitude for the efforts on his part which have led to such a magnificent result. . . . ," the chairman read into the minutes.

As soon as Pasteur's paper was published, people who had been bitten by mad dogs flocked from all sides to his laboratory for treatment. Out of three hundred patients whom he treated, personally arranging for their care during their stay in Paris, all but one had been saved. The little girl, whose death caused Pasteur to burst into tears as he saw her breathe her last, had been brought to him thirty-seven days after she was bitten. Too late!

Then came the nineteen Russians who had been attacked by a rabid wolf. Accompanied by a Russian doctor they travelled all the way from the province of Smolensk. Because they were in such bad condition on their arrival, Pasteur decided on two inoculations a day. A fortnight had passed between the time they were bitten and the first inoculation. Eighty-two out of

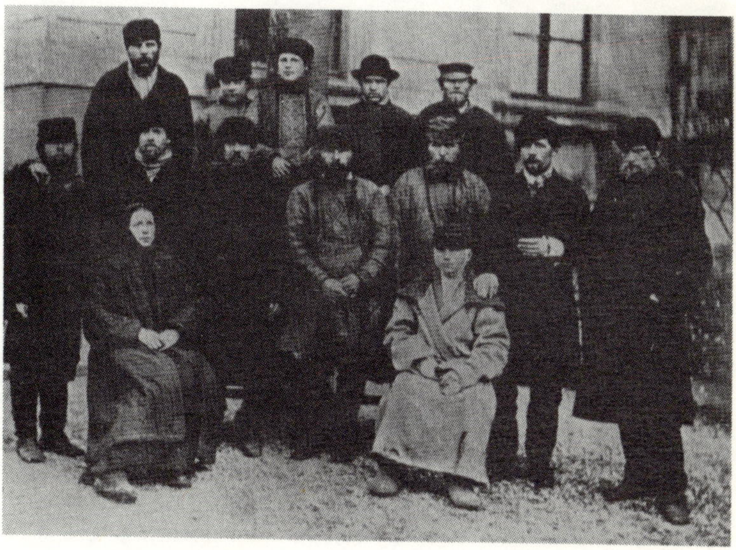

Russians from Smolensk who were among the first to receive injections against wounds inflicted by a wolf with rabies

every hundred had, previously, been known to die from rabid wolf bites. The world awaited the outcome, and received the news of the death of three of the Russian peasants with grief. The remaining sixteen returned to their country without having contracted rabies. The Czar sent an Imperial gift, the Cross of the Order of St. Anne, set in diamonds. Besides, he added 100,000 francs for the proposed Pasteur Institute.

Pasteur's last years were far from serene. The ignorant and the envious lost not a single opportunity to criticize and slander,

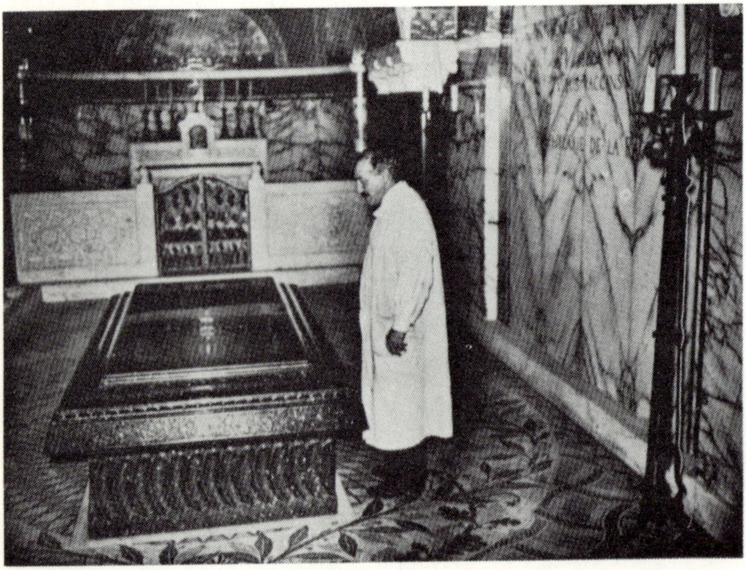

The first man to have received an injection against rabies visits Pasteur's tomb in the Pasteur Institute in Paris on the 50th anniversary of Pasteur's death

to insinuate that he had failed to report the accidents and failures. To the end he was forced into defensive debates.

Remembered by his grandson, himself a distinguished physician and scientist, "as a very simple and very kind man," in the waning years of his life, paralyzed, and his strength failing, he spent his summers at Villeneuve l'Etang, near the Kennels.

On the holidays he took at Arbois, "Sometimes a wine grower, his basket on his back, stopped when he saw him, called him Louis, and addressed him in a familiar way. Was he not a son of this region? Those who went by him on the road without knowing him did not think that such a simple and modest man could be Pasteur!"

While at times he confided to the boy that if he had his life over again, he would undertake again his studies on crystals, his grandson remembers that more often he would say: "I am convinced that science and peace will triumph over ignorance and war."

6

THE DOCTOR'S WANDERLUST FULFILLED

Koch Continues

JUST ABOUT the time when anthrax had been conquered, Asiatic cholera, which Europeans smugly thought was only an Indian pestilence, suddenly struck at the eastern edge of the continent. One of the worst epidemics gripped the people of Egypt. Alexandria was a city of death. No one knew who would be the next victim of agonizing cramps and spasms and within a day be counted among the hundreds of dead. The people in Central Europe were stricken with fear. If the plague could travel over the Indian Ocean and the Asiatic desert, how long would it be before it would cross the Mediterranean Sea?

It was then that the German Government sent Koch to Egypt to search out the threatening invisible enemy. Koch packed his microscope and his collection of animals and, with Gaffky, took the next train from Berlin.

In Paris, Pasteur had to make the painful choice between setting out on such an expedition to the East, and continuing with his work on rabies at home. He proposed to the Committee of Public Hygiene that they send a French Scientific Mission.

"What is wanted at this moment . . . is to inquire into the

primary cause of the scourge. Now the present state of knowledge demands that attention should be drawn to the possible existence within the blood, or within some organ, of a microorganism . . . The proved existence of such a microbe would soon take precedence over the whole question of the measures to be taken to arrest the evil in its course, and might perhaps suggest new methods of treatment."

The Committee approved the plan and asked him to choose some young men for the project. Roux immediately offered to go. Two older men who qualified by their training and work in the laboratory also volunteered, while young Thuillier said he would like twenty-four hours to think about it. It was

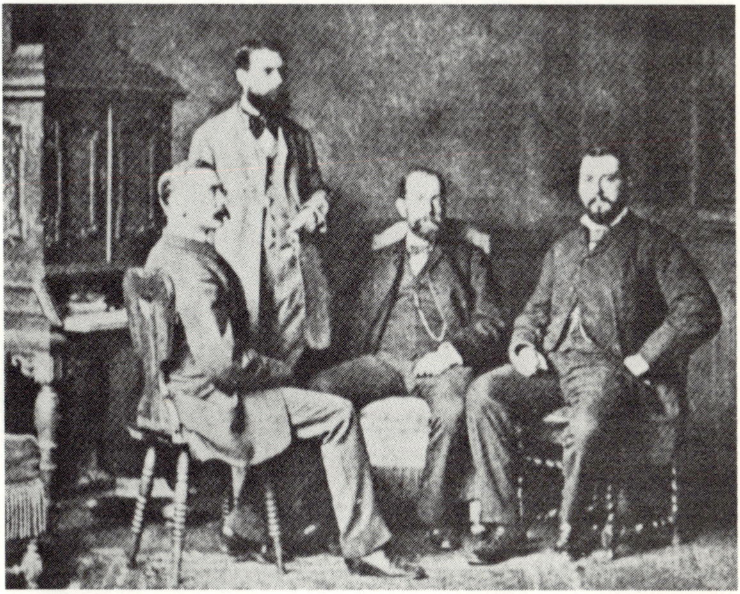

Robert Koch (seated centre) and his assistants during the cholera epidemic of 1883. Seated at Koch's left is von Behring; at his right is Loeffler. The man standing is probably Gaffky

not for himself that he had any hesitation, but for his father and mother who had made a great many sacrifices to send him to school. "You are not going to Egypt, Louis; swear that you are not," his older sister cried. "I am not going to swear anything," he announced calmly. He had made up his mind.

The German and the French teams worked separately. Partly out of nationalistic feeling and partly because of personal animosity between Koch and Pasteur, the two groups in quest of a deadly enemy carried on the work as if they were racing with each other.

In the miserable hospitals and morgues they performed autopsies on the dead Egyptians, examining the contents of the intestines. There they found a variety of microbes, but which was the one that caused cholera? They worked at preparing different cultures to shoot into cats, dogs, swine, guinea-pigs, rabbits, monkeys, and pigeons, but each time the results were negative. They were making no headway in their attempts to reproduce the disease in animals. Just then, as suddenly as it came, the epidemic mysteriously disappeared. All their work was for the moment in vain, and Koch and Gaffky were preparing to leave for home.

Then the dreadful news came that Thuillier had succumbed to cholera and died. The two Germans were as shaken as the French Commission. As Emile Roux reported: "M. Koch and his collaborators arrived when the news spread in the town. When the funeral took place, those gentlemen brought two wreaths which they themselves nailed on the coffin. 'They are simple,' said M. Koch, 'but they are of laurel, such as are given to the brave.' M. Koch held one corner of the pall."

The death of a battler in a common cause weighed heavily on the German who returned to Berlin without further delay. He had found a germ, stained it, and discovered that its shape was like a comma. He was anxious to report this discovery to the Minister of State, but he said that he hadn't yet proved that this was the deadly cause of cholera. He begged to be sent to India where cholera was ever lurking. He was sure he was on the right track, but had to follow it to its end.

Koch then sailed for Calcutta with his mice and microscope and bottles of stains, a curious figure on a strange mission. After months at sea and suffering from seasickness, he was in India.

In dozens of dead bodies and in the intestines of patients sick with cholera, he found the comma bacillus, a fine curved little stick, which he never saw in healthy persons or in any of the animals he examined. The next step was to grow the germ pure. He was by now a past master at cultivating microbes and soon found he could grow the cholera spirillum on beef-broth jelly. Next he studied its ways, and discovered that it died the moment it was dried, while it lived in the open cisterns from which the Hindus got their foul drinking water. This was the way it invaded the healthy body. After that it easily spread from the sick to the healthy through soiled bed-linen and the clothing of those who had perished.

His mission completed, Koch returned to Germany, where the news of his discovery had preceded him. No military hero was ever received with greater honours. The German Emperor himself presented the one-time village doctor with the Order of the Crown. In the simple way in which he had once demonstrated his capture of the anthrax bacillus, he now told the Berlin doctors that "cholera never rises spontaneously." Cholera attacks only those who swallow the comma bacillus; "it cannot be produced from any other thing, or out of nothing . . . it is only in the intestine of man, or in highly polluted water . . . that it can grow."

If cholera outbreaks still recur with frightening regularity in the Far East it is because sanitation methods there, even today, are far behind those in other parts of the world.

Koch's pursuit of the cholera bacillus only temporarily interrupted his researches in tuberculosis. When, in 1885, he was appointed Professor of Hygiene and Director of the Hygienic Institute at the University of Berlin, he returned to the work for which he is best known, and which also caused him a great deal of sadness. The cure for the disease which he laboured for over two decades to find eluded him. His attempt to prepare a vaccine brought heartbreaking disappointments.

From cultures of tubercle bacilli he extracted tuberculin, a substance he believed to be a vaccine. There was great excitement when in 1890, at the Tenth International Medical Congress held in Berlin, Koch announced that he had succeeded in isolating a substance which could "check the growth of tubercle bacilli, not only in a test-tube, but also in the animal body."

Fresh hope was held out to consumptive sufferers, and patients flocked from all over the world to try the new remedy. But many met their death because tuberculin did not behave as a vaccine. Koch's announcement was perhaps premature. It is even said that he was under pressure from the authorities to "produce a cure."

While in a normal person tuberculin is comparatively harmless, in a sensitized person it produces a marked reaction. In Koch's consumptive patients tuberculin caused a flare-up of the malady and, in some instances, death. People turned away from his remedy, which was soon discarded.

Over three-quarters of a century has passed since Koch's failure to produce an anti-tubercular vaccine. However, while tuberculin failed to fulfil its discoverer's hopes of a cure, his work opened up new fields of inquiry into the secrets of immunity. Tuberculin, itself modified in different ways and used in small quantities, sometimes has healing qualities. It also has value in the detection of tuberculosis. Some of these fruits of his work Koch lived to see.

During the early years of the twentieth century two Frenchmen, Doctors Calmette and Guerin, developed the now widely used vaccine BCG—Bacillus Calmette-Guerin. This is an attenuated strain of bovine tubercle bacilli produced by successive subculturing so that it becomes avirulent and incapable of producing the disease in humans, but will nevertheless cause the blood to produce protective antibodies.

BCG together with improved standards of housing, working conditions and environmental hygiene has helped in reducing tuberculosis to the rare disease it is today in many countries of the world.

Wholly devoted to research, Koch decided that neither the life of a teacher of hygiene, nor that of a country doctor, was for him. He could not hear of an epidemic anywhere in the world without wanting to take the first train or boat to study it. So he resigned his professorship.

In 1891 he was appointed chief of the newly built Institute for Infectious Diseases which was called by his name. He surrounded himself with able young men from different parts of the world, and extended the results of his fruitful methods. When his pupils returned to their own countries they carried their great master's teachings to their own laboratories, and themselves made brilliant contributions.

As director he could also freely carry on the specialized researches which often took him to many parts of the wide world. Koch set up temporary field laboratories in various tropical regions where many of the destructive epidemics flourished.

Malaria took him to East Africa, Italy, and Java. By learning the life cycle of the parasite he helped to establish a method of prevention. Then the British Government invited him to colonial South Africa to do something about rinderpest, the widespread pestilence of cattle. Off he went to the British colony. Without discovering the cause, he found a means of completely stopping the spread of this destructive cattle plague.

Then his own government sent him to German East Africa to investigate sleeping sickness. He found that where the tsetse fly flourishes sleeping sickness does also, but not where the fly is absent.

In East Africa he discovered a way in which other diseases spread: a variety of blood-sucking ticks through successive generations of infected eggs transmitted disease to humans. A species of tick carrying the infecting spiral-shaped organism caused East African tick fever; other ticks caused Texas fever, a blight in cattle. In the jungle of Africa he transferred from man to ape the organism responsible for relapsing fever. By these discoveries Koch opened a new field of study—tropical microbiology.

Sometimes he directed the searches of his pupils from afar. When, in 1894, Kitasato was sent from Japan to Hong Kong to study the plague, he found the bubonic plague bacilli in infected glands and in the blood of the patient's heart. The erstwhile student, now on his own, cabled the news to Koch.

"Did you succeed in cultivating the bacillus artificially?" the master cabled back.

"Yes," came the answer two days later.

Koch's rules for microbe searches had been followed precisely: mice were inoculated with the blood from the spleen of patients sick with plague, and cultures were made from the animals' blood. The cultures were then shot into guinea pigs and rabbits which died from the infection.

In 1904, the one-time country doctor resigned from his post at the Institute he made famous. Georg Theodor Gaffky, his brilliant pupil, could now replace him as chief. In the dozen years that Koch had held the post, his assistants discovered the causes of no fewer than ten human diseases. He could well entrust future searching to them. But his own interest never waned. Tuberculosis was still the malady that occupied him most, and it was his work on that disease that earned him the 1905 Nobel Prize for Physiology and Medicine. In 1908 he went to America to attend the International Tuberculosis Congress held in Washington.

By then he was 65, but youthful enough to undertake an even longer journey to Japan. The main purpose of this trip was to visit Kitasato, one of his favourite pupils, who was a director of an Institute for Infectious Diseases in Tokyo.

As Koch walked down the gangplank, he seemed tall and spry in his black suit and black bowler hat to the stocky, round-faced Japanese scientist. Under the hat his bald head, "flat on top, and very well developed on the sides," reminded the adoring student of Confucius.

Robert Koch spent forty happy days visiting, being entertained in imperial style by the Japanese scientists who worshipfully called him "Father." The German gloried as much in the remarkable successes of his pupil as if he had been a beloved son who had exceeded his father's fondest hopes.

Koch was in the habit of cutting his own hair, or what was left of it. It is recorded as a fact that Kitasato saved these precious strands, and after Koch's death placed them in the shrine he built for him at the Tokyo Institute.

Nor was Kitasato the only one of his admiring students. Years later Paul Ehrlich, another of his brilliant scientific sons, said of his stay in Koch's laboratory, "This was perhaps the most interesting time of my life."

Koch lived for his work; through his devoted students his work went on after him. To the end of his days he remained the simple, modest searcher for new facts, facts on which to build a science of medicine. Of his many discoveries he said simply: "I came in my wanderings through the medical field upon regions where the gold was still lying by the wayside."

One day in the spring of 1910, Robert Koch died suddenly at Baden-Baden. According to his will his remains were cremated. Only twenty-one persons paid the last honours with a few wreaths. Among the mourners were Frau Koch, Gaffky, Ehrlich, and the Mayor of Baden-Baden. A marble mausoleum in the Koch Institute contains the urn where his ashes were laid to rest. He died as simply as he had lived. This was his desire. No monument could have been more imposing than his work.

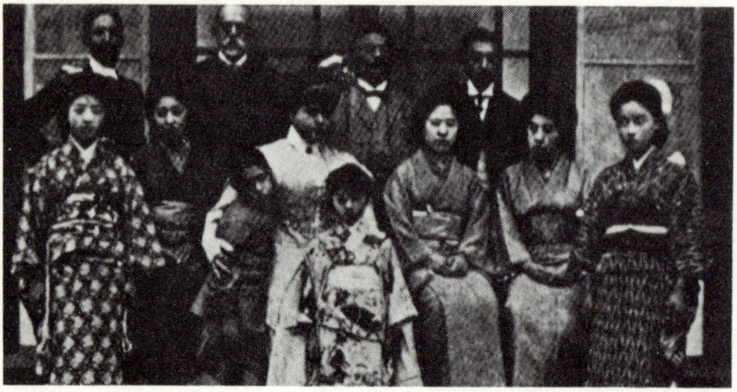

Robert Koch in Japan. At his left is Dr. Kitasato

7

DISCIPLES

IN THE eighteen-eighties, Berlin and Paris were the world's centres of microbiology and Koch and Pasteur the undisputed masters. The institutes directed by Pasteur, the visionary, and Koch, the master of method, were buzzing with the exciting search for new murderous germs. From every part of Europe, America, and Japan, eager students converged upon these laboratory centres, and became disciples of the great founders of the new science.

In the heat of battle against anthrax and cholera, the master bacteriologists sometimes forgot that they were fighting a common enemy. Pasteur and Koch, especially when both had achieved world renown, hated each other. Misdirected patriots were egging each on in the race for glory, in the name of La Patrie and the Vaterland. While the generals were nursing personal grudges, the younger men whom they led in the quest for deadly microbes seemed less inclined to carry on either the private or nationalistic feud. In the war against diphtheria, the deadliest of children's diseases, the engagements crossed national barriers.

The advance operations took place in Koch's laboratory.

Friedrich Loeffler, Koch's lieutenant during the latter's attack on the tubercle bacillus, had done his own spying through the microscope. He was only nine years younger than Koch, and when he had decided on a career as a laboratory scientist, he had already spent some years in the service of the German army as surgeon.

By 1882, in Koch's institute, Loeffler had chalked up two victories in his own name. He had discovered the erysipelas germ in pigs, and from the nasal discharges of horses and mules sick with glanders, a disease that is fatal in half the animals and men who contract it, he isolated the frail but highly poisonous bacillus.

He next turned to diphtheria which, in the severe epidemics stalking all of Europe, was claiming the lives of young children. There was little the doctors could do to save the victims from suffocation, except to pierce the membrane that blocked their windpipe or to cut into that tube. The children's wards rang with the croupy metallic coughs that failed to open the choked-up little throats. One out of every two children struck with the disease turned blue for want of air and died of suffocation as surely as if he had been strangled in a noose. Mothers implored the doctors to save their children, but the healers were powerless.

While studying the grayish-white membrane taken from the throat of a diphtheria patient, Edwin Klebs, a German physician, found the germ. Loeffler, seeing that he could do nothing for the sick, decided he would try to find out from the dead how to conquer the killer. In the morgue of the hospital he went to work with the tools of the microbe searcher: sterile knives, heated platinum wires, broth-filled test-tubes, bottles of dyes, and his microscope. From the grayish stuff that plugged the once living throats he scraped up a bit to put into

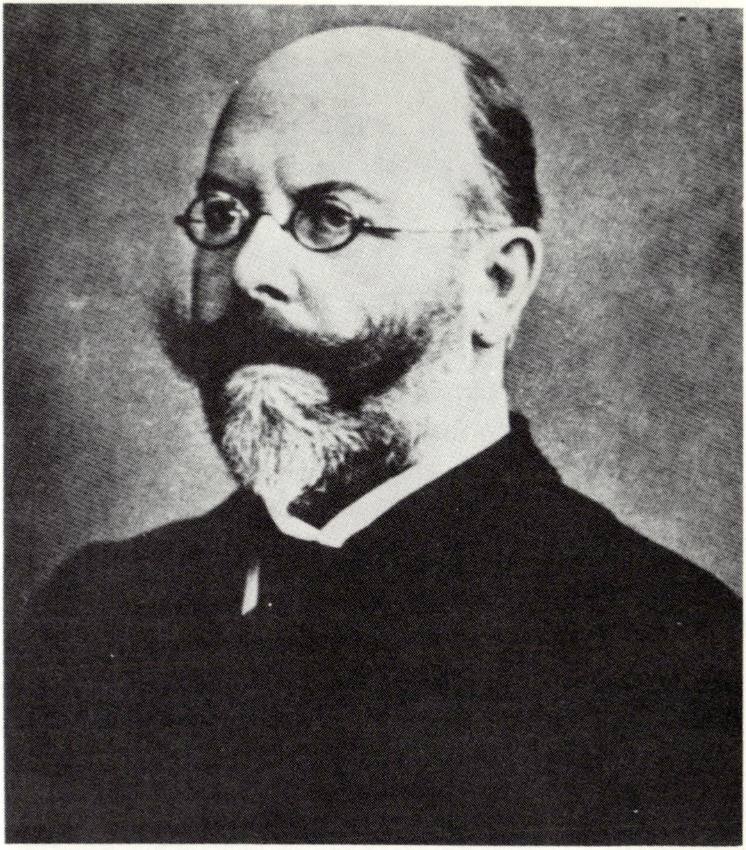

Friedrich Loeffler

his tubes, later to be incubated. Some of it he spread on a thin glass slide, which he heated over an alcohol flame, then dyed with a stain. Through his microscope he saw bacilli shaped like Indian clubs. In nearly every throat of the disease-choked children he saw the same unmistakable bacilli. He rushed to the laboratory to show Koch what he had discovered. Are these little clubs the culprits?

During his training, Loeffler had been warned many times by his patient master never to be sure until all the proof was in, so he guessed what Koch would say. He knew what he had to do, for up to now he had only the clue, which would have to be carried through the well-known steps. With military precision he followed the rules: grow the microbes pure; produce the disease in animals—exactly as it was in the human body; find the same bacilli in the sick animals; with cultures of these, produce the disease in other animals.

He had no trouble in growing the "Indian clubs" pure. (Eventually, these came to be called the Klebs-Loeffler bacilli.) But unlike the anthrax and tubercle bacilli, the disease producers in this case were not to be found in the blood or in any other part of the body. In vain he searched for the bacillus in hundreds of sections from every tissue, but the Indian clubs seemed to have made their haven only in the choked-up throats. Strange, that the small number of germs concentrated in one tiny spot should have killed a child within a few days! Loeffler puzzled over this, but could not find an explanation. At any rate, he would have to go on to the next step.

He shot his pure cultivations into the windpipes of rabbits and under the skin of guinea pigs. The animals fell ill and died as the children had. The same curious thing happened here: the germs remained in the spot where they were injected —and nowhere else. Loeffler was stumped. If these germs caused diphtheria, he couldn't prove it beyond a doubt. So he wrote down what he saw, and ended his report with a question mark and conjecture. The bacillus stays in the little spot in the throat of a child. It remains under the skin of the guinea pig. It never grows in millions, nor spreads through the blood. But always it kills. Loeffler couldn't say why. And it didn't paralyze his rabbits as it did the children.

Even more confusing was the fact that sometimes he couldn't find the bacillus in a child who died of diphtheria; on the other hand, once in a while he found it in a healthy child. Why was it that the germ which occasionally was harmless in a child would kill a rabbit? He could hardly know at that time that once in a great while a child who carries the germ may be immune.

Loeffler admitted defeat. Without realizing how close he was to a solution, he ventured a guess, which turned out to be a telling clue for others: The bacillus must brew a poison which leaks out of it into the tissues. This deadly toxin must be found somewhere in the dead child, or in the broth in which it grows in a test tube. "Whoever finds this toxin will prove what I have failed to show," he concluded.

Emile Pierre Paul Roux was born in Confolens, Charente, France, in 1853, one year after Loeffler. His father was the principal of the school he attended.

Later, in medical school, he had the good fortune to study under the distinguished chemist Duclaux who took an interest in him. When his teacher was invited to fill a chair at the Agricultural Institute in Paris, he took Roux with him. Duclaux did him one more good turn when, in 1878, he introduced him to Louis Pasteur. The young physician thus came under the spell of Pasteur's irresistible teachings.

Trained for the profession of medicine, Roux was willing to set aside practical doctoring for what was at first the tedium of laboratory glass-washing. As an assistant in Pasteur's laboratory he had to sterilize tubes and syringes, prepare soups for culturing bacteria, jab needles into guinea pigs, lay the little

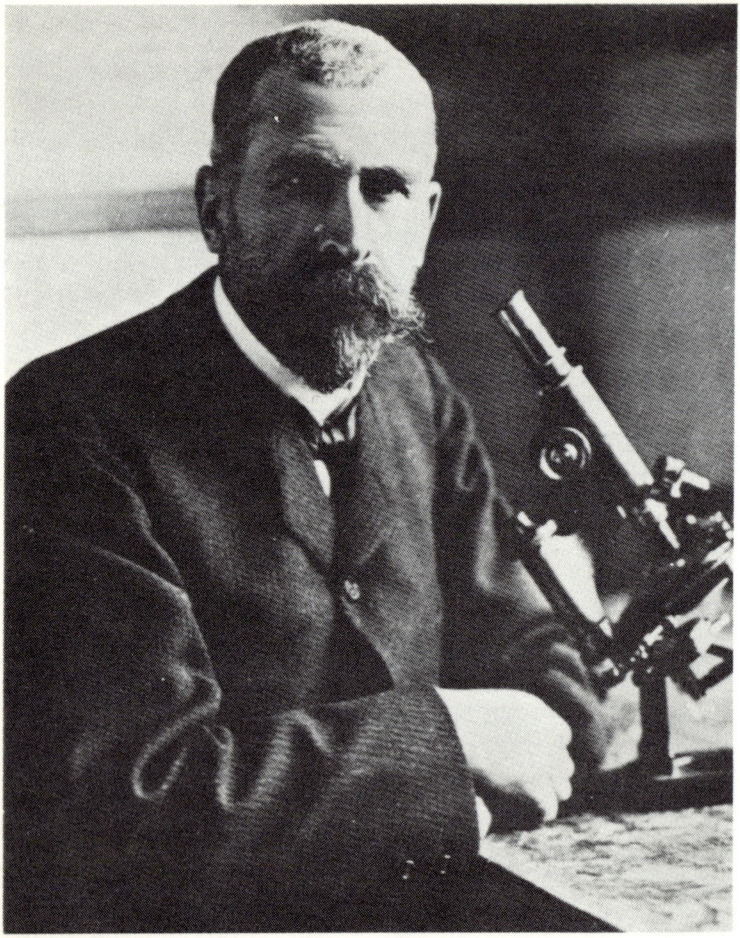

Emile Roux

bodies out on dissecting tables, and clean up after these messy operations. What could have induced him to turn away from the art of healing and become a laboratory drudge?

The truth is that he had little faith in his ability as a healer. Medicine had not advanced beyond prescribing old-fashioned remedies for reducing a fever, clearing up a case of worms, applying poultices to boils and toothaches, and helping to bring babies into the world. If mothers got child-bed fever, and their babies infant diarrhea, if epidemics of typhoid, diphtheria, or plague raged, the doctor was helpless. Pasteur's prophecy that "it is within the power of man to cause all parasitic diseases to disappear from the world" captured the imagination of the young doctor. Along with other eager students, he sat at Pasteur's feet, and became convinced that the conquest of disease meant warfare against wriggling bugs revealed by his microscope.

In the battle with anthrax he had learned how this enemy could be weakened to the point where it could no longer attack. In fact, its weakness became the strength of the patient to fight off the invasion of a deadly bug. Pasteur's methods put powerful tools into the doctor's hands. In Pasteur's laboratory Emile Roux learned the way to weaken microorganisms by drying them as in rabies and aging them as in chicken cholera. He would find still other ways of taming them.

In 1882, he and Charles Edouard Chamberland, another bright medical youngster, struck out on their own and found a way to attenuate or weaken germs with chemicals. Still alive, but their virulence crippled, the little killers no longer poisoned, but instead built the animal's defences against further attacks.

Five years after Loeffler's discovery of the diphtheria bacillus, children were still dying from that dreaded disease. A mother wrote to Pasteur:

"You have done all the good a man could do on earth. If you will, you can surely find a remedy for the horrible disease called diphtheria. Our children, to whom we teach your name as that of a great benefactor, will owe their lives to you."

It was an open letter to all desperate searchers for a cure.

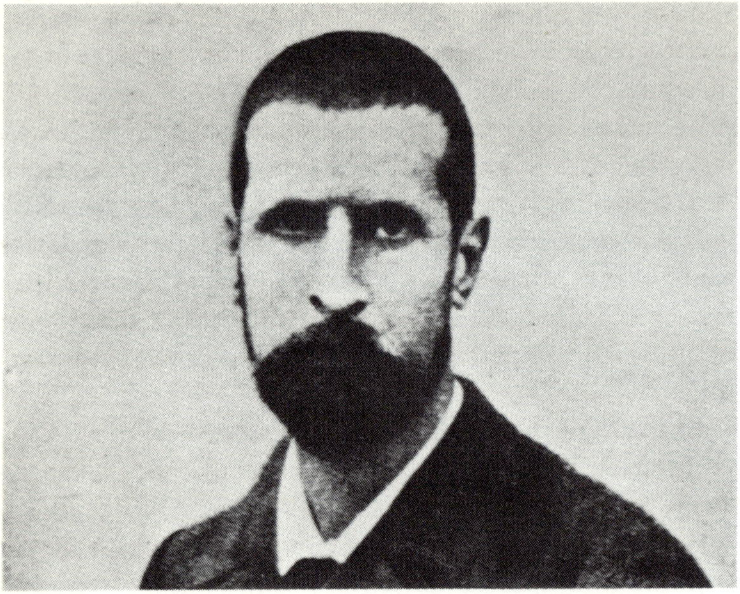

Alexandre Yersin

This time, with Alexandre Yersin, a Swiss student from Lausanne, who joined the Pasteur crusaders, Roux tackled the problem anew. Yersin was ten years younger than Roux, and this was a splendid opportunity to work with a brilliant pupil of the great master. In the Hospital for Sick Children, they went after the germs which settled in the throats of diphtheritic babies. Here they picked up the same bacillus the German had described earlier.

They began by growing the Indian clubs in flasks of veal broth, and shot the cultures into birds and all kinds of laboratory animals. They followed in Loeffler's footsteps, but they didn't reach the same dead end. Perhaps it was luck, but Roux' and Yersin's rabbits did show the telling paralysis. This provided the proof Loeffler was unable to get—the disease was the same as in children. On to the next step. If this bacillus *was* the true cause of diphtheria, they would search for it in the tissues.

They were no more successful than Loeffler. The French investigators were faced with the same big question mark. What killed their animals, if the bugs were nowhere to be seen in the thousands of tissue slices they examined? It was then that Roux remembered Loeffler's words: "whoever finds this toxin . . ." Could it be that the Indian clubs manufacture a poison which trickles across the delicate walls of the tiniest blood vessels? Is it this toxin circulating in the veins that kills? This was a brand new thought, for no one had yet separated the poison from the bodies of germs. But how would they go about proving it?

"To begin with," Roux argued, "if the bacilli form a toxin in the throat membrane which they pour into the blood, they must also make it in the broth in which we grow them."

The next step would then be to separate the poison from the culture. For this they devised the finest of filters—a porcelain tube with pores so fine that they would let the broth through but hold back the bacilli. But the scientists outdid themselves—the sieve was too close-meshed to let even the soup through. Persisting in their determination to make the separation, they used a suction system, until a clear filtered fluid came through without a germ in it. If this stuff contained toxin, it should kill the animals.

The logic was clear, but when they shot fluid into the veins of guinea pigs they waited in vain for signs of illness. They kept increasing the dose and repeating the injections, but the animals were as frisky as ever. Still Roux wouldn't give up, so convinced was he that the soup must contain the toxin. With the stubbornness of a Pasteur he persisted until he finally shot a whole test-tubeful of the stuff under the skin of his animals, and then he reproduced the disease. Like the ones that had received the live bacilli, the guinea pigs choked for breath and died within several days. In this way Roux proved that the symptoms of diphtheria were due to the toxin made by the bacilli.

It was months later that he discovered why the filtered toxin he used was so weak. He had not incubated his cultures long enough. When he left his germ-filled tubes in the incubator for six weeks instead of four days, the toxin became so concentrated that even the smallest drop would work havoc with his animals. A single ounce of the concentrated poison was enough to kill six hundred thousand guinea pigs.

The next step was to find a way to prevent the germs from making the toxin—the only way to protect babies against diphtheria. But for this part of our story we travel back to Germany.

In the year when Roux and Yersin discovered the diphtheria toxin, Emil von Behring, then thirty-five-years old, came to work as an assistant in Koch's institute. Born in West Prussia, he entered the Military Medical Academy at Berlin at twenty. Upon graduation he joined the Army Medical Corps, becoming a lecturer at the Army Medical College in 1888. His heart seemed to be in research, however, so a year later he joined the young men in the famous Koch laboratory, where he met Kitasato who had preceded him there by four years.

Shibasaburo Kitasato, sent by the Japanese Government, came to Berlin shortly after Koch returned from India after his discovery of the cholera vibrio, so called because it was capable of spontaneous movement. It was a great honour to be sponsored by his government, for which the young man risked

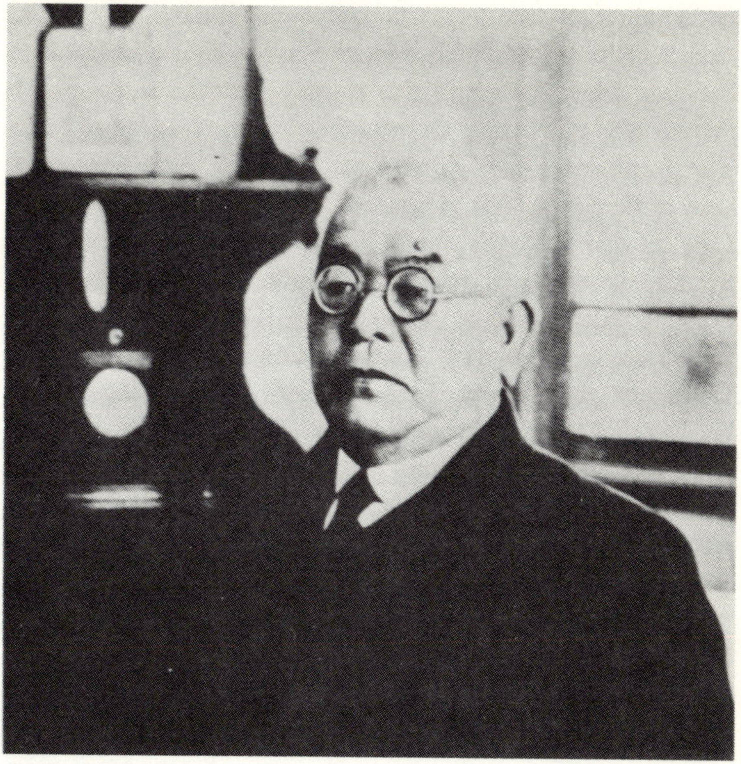

Shibasaburo Kitasato

a two months' journey through the Indian Ocean, as a steerage passenger. But to Kitasato, the greatest honour was the privilege of working with the "Father of Bacteriology."

Kitasato was born in 1852 in Ogiungo, a mountain village in the south of Japan. His father was a knight under the feudal system of Japan. He sent the boy to the newly established medical school in Kumamoto, where he studied under the European Professor Mansfield. From there he went on to the government medical school in Tokyo, and after completing his studies he joined the Public Health Service. This was just about the time when the world was ringing with the discoveries of Pasteur and Koch, and the echoes were heard as far as Japan. The government singled out Kitasato as one of the students to send to Berlin. In 1885, he arrived at Koch's Hygiene Institute. Like the rest of Koch's pupils, he was put through the rigorous training in the bacteriologic techniques and methods of the exacting teacher.

Within a short time Kitasato showed his talents in the laboratory and was assigned the task of searching for the bacillus that causes tetanus, or lockjaw. Kitasato knew the gruesome disease that sometimes throws every muscle into a taut spasm, distorting the facial muscles as the victim exerts a painful effort to open the jaw. In agonizing pain, the patient fairly jumps at the slightest noise or touch.

In isolating the germ, Kitasato discovered the tetanus bacillus, one of a group of *anaerobic* bacteria, which can live without air.

"I could not believe my eyes," Koch said, "when he showed me the gelatin medium in which the tetanus bacilli had grown, because such trained and experienced scholars as Gaffky and Loeffler had not yet succeeded in the experiment so easily carried out by Kitasato. I could not overcome my surprise for a time, and realized that the small Japanese figure had indeed the power and talent to solve the difficult problem of obtaining a pure culture of the tetanus bacillus. I immediately ordered him to try animal experiments with the bacillus he had isolated and to watch for the symptoms to develop. . . . Imagine the joy I experienced when I was convinced of every detail in his success."

As Kitasato got to know the tetanus bug better, he found

that like the diphtheria bacillus it produced a toxin which it cast off into the blood. He injected the lockjaw cultures into the tails of mice, and then cut them off. Even without their infected tails, the mice died from the poison that was circulating in their blood. Thus he discovered the tetanus toxin, and like Roux, showed that some bacteria kill by the poison they give off.

At this point (1890) von Behring joined Kitasato in the battle against tetanus. Together they found that they could make an animal immune to lockjaw. By injecting it with blood serum from an animal that had been infected with tetanus, they could protect it against the disease. Even when they shot 300 times the fatal dose of tetanus toxin into its tissues, the rabbit would still be protected by the antitoxic serum. They published their report, in which for the first time the word "antitoxin" was used. This was a brand new idea—an antidote for a toxin produced by bacteria! For the deadliest of poisons—one-four-thousandth of a gram kills a man—they had discovered a natural antidote, tetanus antitoxin.

One would have thought that since von Behring was one step ahead of Roux, he could pick up from where the Frenchman had left off, and go on to the discovery of a diphtheria antitoxin. But he took a detour on the path to this discovery.

Von Behring thought he could cure diphtheria with powerful chemicals—chemicals that would kill the bugs but be harmless to animals and people. He shot virulent diphtheria bacilli into guinea pigs, and then tried to cure the sick little beasts with different chemicals, experimenting with one after another, including salts of gold. But whether from diphtheria or from the chemicals that he squirted under their skin, the animals died.

Then one day a few guinea pigs that had received both the

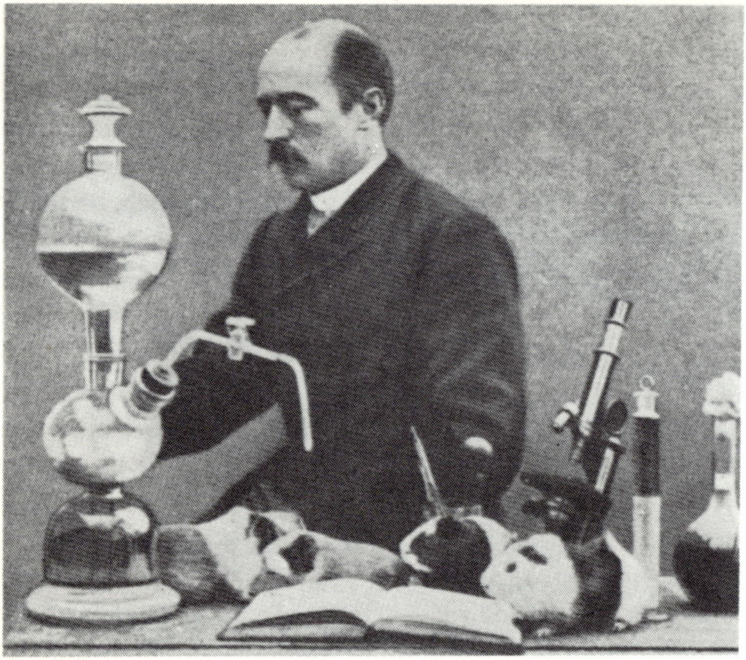

Emil von Behring

deadly dose of diphtheria germs and a chemical containing iodine, miraculously survived the ordeal. When they should have been stretched out dead, they were somehow getting better.

Von Behring was sure he had now found a cure for diphtheria. But when he continued with this experiment of making the animals sick and then trying the "cure," they died just as often from the iodine trichloride, which ate holes in their skins, as from the disease.

Still, now and then, some animals recovered from diphtheria. What would happen if he gave these cured guinea pigs another dose of diphtheria bacilli? Imagine his astonishment when ten times the ordinary dose hardly upset them. They were immune!

It was then that von Behring realized that he had been on the wrong path with the chemical cure. There must be something in the blood that worked the cure. He had always thought that there was no end to the remarkable things the life-stream could do! To find out what it was he planned another kind of experiment.

He drew some blood from the cured guinea pigs, and let it stand in tubes until the clear-coloured serum separated from the solid part of the blood. Then he added this serum to a flask containing virulent diphtheria organisms. He fully expected that the serum would kill the microbes. But there they were on his slide, alive under his microscope. In fact they were multiplying, growing luxuriantly.

Here von Behring turned to Emile Roux' results. It was the diphtheria toxin, and not the bacilli, that was deadly. He would go back to his cured animals; only this time he would inject them with the poison brewed by the microbes. Sure enough, they were immune to the toxin, as they were to the live bacilli.

The antidote must be in the blood. He was certain that that's where he would have to look for it. So he drew some blood from his cured animals, hoping and praying that he would succeed in getting enough of this precious stuff from his convalescing guinea pigs. He mixed the few drops of serum he collected with some diphtheria toxin taken from a tube in which the diphtheria bacilli were grown, and he was ready for the final experiment.

He shot the mixture into new guinea pigs that had not had the disease, and waited and watched. They too remained alive and healthy! So it *was* the blood serum that contained the antidote! The toxin *along with the antitoxin* was as harmless as salt water. But was it really serum, any serum, or only that of cured animals? If Behring had not asked this question himself, you may be sure that someone in that laboratory trained under the great Koch would have asked it. The proof was not yet complete.

Von Behring repeated the experiment, this time mixing toxin and serum taken from a non-immune animal. A syringeful of the mixture was tried on guinea pigs that never had the disease. Within a couple of days all the familiar symptoms appeared—the fever, the cough, the laboured breath, and then they were dead.

The conclusion was clear. "Only serum of immune animals —those which had had diphtheria and were cured—contained the antidote to the diphtheria toxin," von Behring recorded.

The experiment was over. The proof was in. Now it was time to put his results to work, to prevent diphtheria. During months of feverish activity, von Behring built up a large supply of the antidote-containing serum.

He started his deadly microbes in his flask on veal soup to produce their poison, and used rabbits, dogs, and sheep to manufacture the healing serum.

He still used the iodine trichloride with the diphtheria toxin which he injected into sheep to make them build up the antitoxin in their blood. He gave them enough of the poison to goad their tissues into producing antitoxin, but not to kill them. When the sheep recovered, their serum contained the protective antitoxin. A tiny dose of this serum protected guinea pigs and rabbits against deadly doses of toxin, but their unprotected litter-mates succumbed and died.

He reversed his experiment—first he shot the filtered poison, made the animals sick, and then gave sheep serum to half of them. It worked. These animals got well, while those which did not receive the serum died.

Just when he thought he could begin to protect children against diphtheria, and the world was full of hope, he found that the protection the antitoxin gave his animals was fleeting. It lasted for a week, two or three at the most, but after that the animals could withstand less and less poison. How practical would it be to jab children with needles every few weeks?

But if a child already had the disease, was perhaps dying, would the serum save its life?

Then came Christmas 1891. A child choking with diphtheria in a hospital bed in Berlin was given the first shot of antitoxin. The child miraculously recovered. Within the next several years thousands of other children were cured with antitoxin. Diphtheria antitoxin proved a success, except that occasionally a child died—died suddenly almost as soon as the serum had been injected. Parents became frightened of a cure that carried such a risk. Some doctors—the inevitable doubters—raised a hue and cry against sheep serum, and so progress against the disease was halted.

In the meantime Emile Roux kept working in his Paris laboratory. He discovered that he could make horses immune to the toxin without upsetting the horses in the least. Their bodies became factories for turning out antitoxin. At weekly intervals they were injected with the deadly stuff. Each time they received more than the previous time until, after two or three months, they could endure nearly one thousand times as much of the toxin as would have originally killed them. Then as much as six quarts of their blood could be taken each month and the serum separated and siphoned off from the clot.

It was in the winter of 1894 when an especially severe epi-

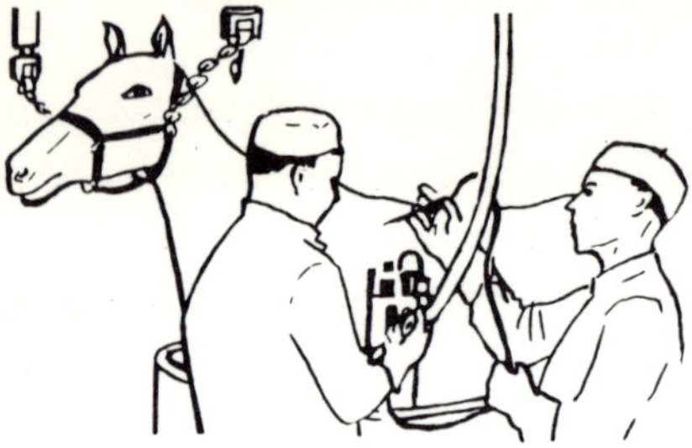

Injecting the dose of toxin

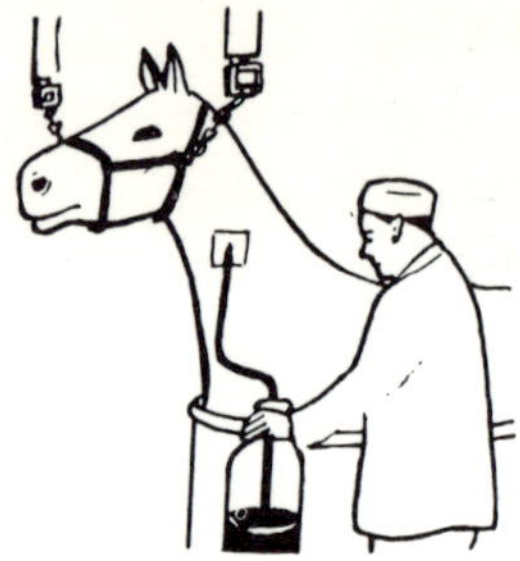

Collecting blood from
immunized animal

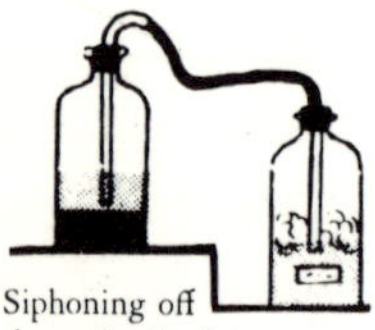

Siphoning off
the antitoxic plasma

(After the solid parts of the blood have settled out, the fluid part is the *serum* which contains the antibodies)

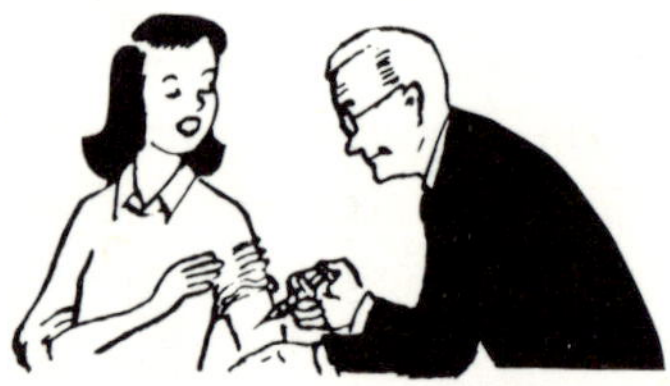

This is injected into the body of a person who needs the antibodies quickly

Diphtheria and tetanus antitoxins are made by the horse when injected either with the bacteria or their toxin

demic gripped Paris. And Roux was ready with the saving serum. During the next few months 300 children received the protective injection and all became well. By the summer, at the International Congress of Medicine held at Budapest, Hungary, Emile Roux was able to tell the world of his healing antitoxin.

The idea that diphtheria could be rendered harmless, perhaps even banished, appealed to the imagination of a world that had mourned the death of many dear ones. A public subscription was arranged for, and the francs began to roll in to the Pasteur Institute for preparation and distribution of the antitoxin.

The Paris Academy of Medicine bestowed a prize of 25,000 francs to Roux and Behring jointly, and the Institute of France followed with a similar prize of 50,000 francs.

Emile Roux returned to his classes in Paris, drawing thousands of students from every quarter of the world. Despite his illness with tuberculosis, which drained his energies, he directed the work of his pupils of all nationalities. In 1895 he was appointed assistant director of the Pasteur Institute, and in 1904 he succeeded his old teacher, Duclaux, as director. By inspiring other researchers as much as by making important contributions himself he continued for many years to uphold the great Pasteur tradition. For many years Roux suffered with chronic tuberculosis; yet he stayed at his post as director of the institute, guiding the work of his followers until his death in 1933.

Kitasato returned to his native land in 1892. The German government bestowed on him the title of "Professor," the first such honour granted by it to a foreign scientist. In his own country he established a laboratory for the study of infectious diseases. Two years later the epidemic of plague broke out in Hong Kong. The world was horrified. The "Black Death" which had killed 70,000 persons in London during 1665 seemed to have been banished, but suddenly, more than two centuries later it hit with renewed vigour in Hong Kong. Japan sent Kitasato to face the attack.

Within two days Kitasato isolated the bacillus of plague from the infected glands of patients who had died from the plague. Then, following in the footsteps of his great teacher, he established it as the cause of the disease which once had swept over Europe and destroyed one-fourth of its population.

Meanwhile Yersin, who had left the Pasteur Institute to make his scientific home in China, arrived in Hong Kong about a week after the Japanese mission. Independently of Kitasato he discovered the bacillus. There was some discussion as to whose description of the organism was correct, but in the end Kitasato agreed that they were both talking about the same plague bacillus.

After their successful campaign against the plague, each returned to his laboratory. There was ample opportunity for Kitasato to pioneer in his own country where he became known as "The Japanese Koch." Under his direction a bacteriological institute developed and prospered. He had a gift for collecting able young men whose talents he helped to develop. He directed research, went abroad on various missions, and during years of strenuous work raised the standards of medical education and public health in Japan. He received many honours abroad, and was also made a baron in his own country.

Throughout his life he never forgot his debt to Koch, whom he loved and worshipped as a hero. At every anniversary of Koch's death, he commemorated the occasion with the appropriate Shinto ceremony at the shrine he built for him in the inner court of his institute.

A great scientist, teacher, and medical leader, Kitasato made an enduring name for himself in medical history.

In his adopted country, Alexandre Yersin prepared a serum to combat the plague. The Chinese Government supported him

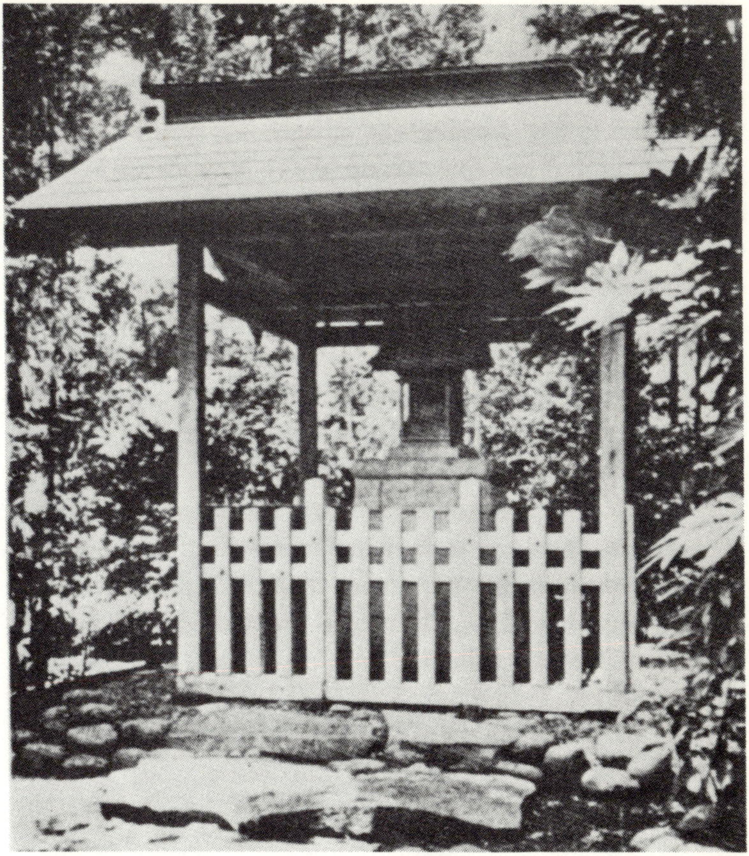

Temple to Koch in Japan, built by Kitasato

in his efforts to set up a branch of the Pasteur Institute at Canton, which he directed. He established a similar institution at Nha Nang Annam to develop bacteriologic research. His work was recognized in Europe, and in 1927 he was awarded the Grand Prize Leconte by the Paris Academy of Sciences. Yersin devoted the major part of his life to improving the health of the people of Indo-China where he died in 1943.

"Not to heal, to prevent," was von Behring's motto for the physician. The work he chose for himself was in keeping with this belief. Partly because of ill health, but chiefly because of his interest in the development of antitoxic sera he gave up his teaching and the directorship at the Institute of Hygiene at Marburg. His desire to manufacture sera led to his connection with a chemical firm where he worked in a lavishly equipped laboratory.

Von Behring was showered with honours by nearly every country of Europe, and by the United States and Mexico. In 1901 he received the first Nobel Prize for his achievements as the most prominent investigator in medicine, and the German Emperor raised him to peerage in 1903.

The academic honours were his own, but the material success of von Behring's large-scale manufacture of antitoxin was in no small measure due to another of Koch's disciples whose life was linked with von Behring's, but who in the light of history left him far behind.

8

DISCIPLE TO CREATOR OF IDEAS

Paul Ehrlich (1854–1915)

In 1876, when Robert Koch went to the University of Breslau to demonstrate his amazing results with the anthrax bacillus, he was shown around the various laboratories. At a bench where a young student was working with bottles of dyes and tissue slices, Koch was told, "This is little Ehrlich. He is very good at staining, but he will *never* pass his examinations."

Neither the doctor, still a long way from world fame, nor the young student listening wide-eyed to Koch's demonstration in Breslau could know that years after this casual meeting they would join hands as collaborators. Dr. Koch returned to his patients and office laboratory and Paul Ehrlich to his bench.

The German chemical works were turning out new aniline dyes. Some of these could stain microscopically thin slices of tissues. Different tissues, their cells, and even parts of cells took on different colours. The dyes became tools for biological work, a way of distinguishing one from the other. During his first college year, spent partly in the University of Strasbourg, Paul Ehrlich became so interested in using these fascinating stains that he often neglected his regular university courses. One day, long after everyone had left the laboratory, Professor Waldeyer found Paul still working at a cluttered table, his hands covered with dyes of all possible colours.

"What do you think you are doing?" Waldeyer asked.

"I am experimenting with dyes," the young man answered without stopping his work.

The professor looked at his stained preparations and soon recognized that the boy was earnestly following his own creative ideas.

"Very well then, keep on; something may come of it," Waldeyer said, and left his student to his work.

Something did come of it. In these experiments, Ehrlich discovered a new type of cell—mast cell, one of the protective white blood cells. By itself, it may have been a minor discovery, but his interest in tissue-staining developed into his life-long idea of using dyes to attach themselves to invading germs and interfere with their growth, without damaging the tissue.

Paul Ehrlich, the only son of an inn-keeper, was born in 1854 in Strehlen, now Eastern Germany. His parents were delighted that their wish for a boy in a household of girls had been fulfilled. Paul's father was a man with his head in the clouds. Though he was the prosperous proprietor of the Tavern of the Wreath of Rue, he contributed hardly more than his good cheer and perhaps also the romantic name to his business establishment. It was Frau Ehrlich who had the burden of attending the inn's guests, supervising the workers, to say nothing of taking wonderful care of the large family. All this she did with skill, wisdom, and good humour.

Paul was said to resemble his grandfather, a kindly, wise, and energetic man whose interest in natural science and in the people of Strehlen found an outlet in the science lectures he gave at the age of eighty. Like his grandfather, little Paul showed an early enthusiasm for nature and, in later years, gave vivid and imaginative explanations of his scientific observations. Often he was so carried away as to earn for himself the nickname of "Doctor Fantasy."

Despite his small build and shy manner his schoolmates at the Strehlen school recognized his leadership. On vacations and holidays, when they played the Silesian version of cops and robbers, Paul organized the games. For who else at the age of eight would have thought of getting the town apothecary to make up cough drops to his own prescriptions? It was Paul who always knew where to catch the most lizards, tadpoles, frogs, and mice. On one occasion he frightened the wits out of the family servant, when she entered the laundry and found the salamanders, frogs, and the rest of pond life escaping from the washtubs where he had left them the night before. To his great disappointment his mother made him return his precious livestock to their natural habitat, and to empty his pockets of insects and worms.

He did well enough in school, especially in Latin and mathematics which he loved, but holidays were always welcome, for then he could throw his books into a corner and occupy himself in other pursuits with his admiring playmates in the hills, woods, or the laundry.

When he was sixteen he went to Breslau College where he lived in the home of his assigned teacher, in a cheerless, bare little room.

Latin and mathematics were easy for him. Both were so logical that they appealed to his well-organized mind. Not so with German composition. He chewed on his pencil, stared at the paper, and tugged at his ear for hours, but the composition remained unwritten. Examinations were even worse. Late into the night he would sit over his books by the light of his paraffin lamp, trying to keep his feet warm at the dying fire in the little stove, and his wandering thoughts on his lessons. One morning, in the examination room, the teacher wrote on the blackboard the subject of the German composition: "Life—A Dream."

Paul Ehrlich was the last to hand in his paper, but even so he had little to show for his distressing efforts. "Now, Paul, would you mind telling me what you mean by this?" the headmaster demanded. "Well, you see," the boy stammered, "life is . . . a . . . chemical incident . . . a normal oxidation . . . and the dream . . . also . . . the dream is . . . the dream is a phosphorescence of the brain."

The teachers and headmaster shrugged their shoulders. Paul's composition was wretchedly bad, a disgrace to the school as well as to himself. But on the strength of his earnestness, and his proficiency in Latin and mathematics, they overlooked his deficiencies. That night Paul was able to send a telegram to his parents which said simply: "Examination passed." And home he went to Strehlen.

In the autumn he returned to Breslau, this time to enter as a university student. His university career was by ordinary standards no more outstanding than his early school years in that institution. He was interested only in biology, the microscopical study of tissues and organic chemistry. After the first term he moved to the University of Strasbourg where Professor Waldeyer gave him his chemical outlook into medicine at a time when little or no chemistry was required of medical students. After a while he returned to Breslau where he had the opportunity to work under Professor Cohnheim, the man who dismissed his classes one day so that they could hear what Koch had to say about anthrax.

Ehrlich finally went on to Leipzig where he graduated as Doctor of Medicine in 1878. His thesis dealt with the value of staining with aniline dyes in the field of medicine. He never ceased experimenting with dyes, some of which he carried on in the little inn where he went for his meals. Years later when he had become famous, the daughter of the inn-keeper wrote to him, reminding him of the time when the towels in the rooms were covered with great spots of dye of every shade that no amount of washing would remove. Even the billiard table, the only one he could use, carried his indelible stains.

After leaving the university he became Assistant and later Senior House Physician at the Charité Hospital in Berlin, where the director was sympathetic to Ehrlich's bent for research. To get to what he called his laboratory, he had to stumble through a dark entrance where the brooms, water pails, and dissecting tables were stored. His laboratory equipment consisted of two pots, dozens of glass vessels and bottles filled with dyes, a Bunsen burner, an incubator, and a water tap. The two pots held his "anatomical collection"—a rare piece of a cancer and a tissue specimen with a chancre, a diseased ulcer.

The director saw to it that Ehrlich's clinical duties were light in order to give the young doctor the freedom he wanted to carry out his experiments. This was a happy, carefree period in his life.

"Karl, a caviar sandwich," was his daily order to the boy who made himself generally useful around the laboratory. But just as regularly the helper would return with a dry bit of ham between two pieces of stale bread. People in the laboratory joked about it and Ehrlich cheerfully replied:

"My dear friends, you don't understand . . . At the moment when I give the order I have at least the pleasure of illusory anticipation: the feeling that it *might* be perhaps, just this once, a caviar sandwich."

The one luxury he permitted himself, and this became a life habit, was the smoking of expensive cigars. He was never without them and, if necessary, would take a cab to the special cigar store to stock up.

In his preoccupation with laboratory work he at no time neglected the patients in the ward. With both infinite skill and the utmost gentleness he carried out procedures which made him a wizard at diagnosing the patient's condition. He became an expert blood-cell stainer, and developed a colour test for urine, a method still helpful in the diagnosis of typhoid fever, measles, and in predicting the outcome in tuberculosis.

Visiting university professors were amazed and impressed with the accuracy and perfection of his work when they saw his crude equipment. "Inspired, simply inspired," the astonished visitor would comment.

It was during the time when Ehrlich was carrying on his fruitful experiments at the Charité Hospital that he married the delightful Hedwig Pinkus, the nineteen-year-old daughter of a wealthy manufacturer in Upper Silesia, and this was also the time when he struck up his friendship with Robert Koch.

Ehrlich attended the meeting of the Physiological Society of Berlin when Koch made a sensation with his announcement of the discovery of the tubercle bacillus in 1882. Ehrlich suddenly remembered that while staining various tissues and sputum from patients with tuberculosis, he had noted rod-shaped bacteria which he did not connect with the disease. Directly after Koch's lecture he hurried to his laboratory to try out his stains on the organism. Since it was late at night, he left his preparations on top of an iron stove to dry. The fire had gone out long before. The next morning the cleaning woman lit the fire in the little stove, paying no attention to the glass slides on it.

When Ehrlich came into the laboratory the next morning and saw the fire in the stove he rushed over, thinking his specimens were lost. But when he added the dye and held the slides up to the light, he saw with delight that they were beautifully stained. Under the microscope it was easy to see the tubercle bacilli in clumps. Ehrlich put this accident down to good luck—the warmth of the stove had intensified the staining process. At once he went to tell Koch what he had discovered. Only twenty-four hours after Koch's reading of his paper on the tubercle bacillus, the master stainer had devised a method for showing up these germs. Koch was the first to recognize the importance of the technique, because he later wrote:

"It was soon found that, with Ehrlich's method of staining, the recognition of tubercle bacilli could readily be made use of in diagnosis. We owe it to this circumstance alone that it has become a general custom to search for the bacillus in sputum, whereas, without it, it is likely that but few investigators would have concerned themselves with tubercle bacilli."

This discovery of Ehrlich was also the occasion for his turning to bacteriology. He became interested in Koch's work of preparing tuberculin.

Just about then, the kindly and indulgent director of the hospital died, and his successor had little use for Ehrlich's experimenting. The atmosphere in the hospital changed so that he found himself stifled. Besides, in 1887, he became ill with tuberculosis which he picked up from his clinic patients.

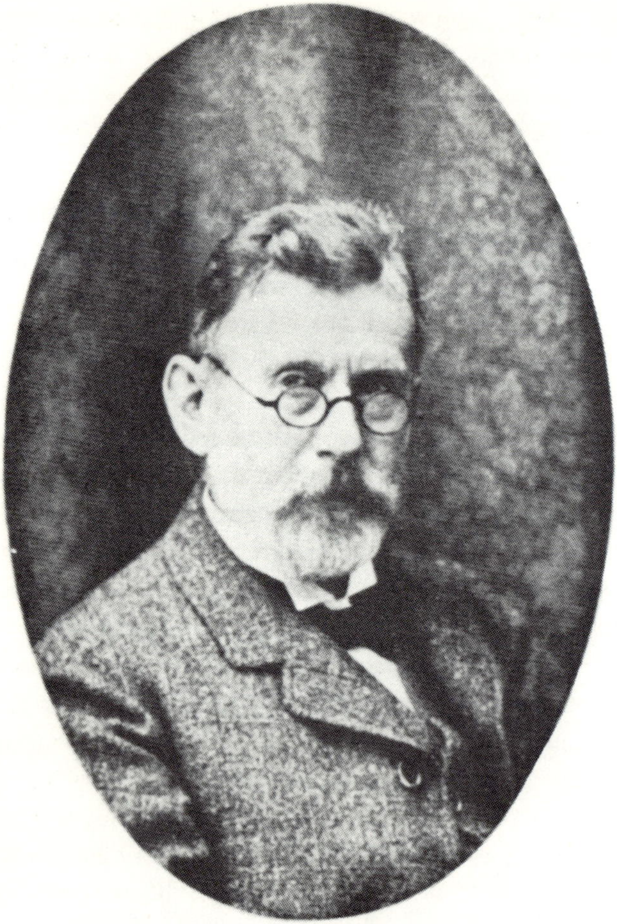

Dr. Paul Ehrlich

Ehrlich resigned from the Charité Hospital and went to Egypt as much to free himself from the rigid routine imposed by the new director as to recover from his lung disease.

When he returned in 1889, he set himself up in a small private laboratory, continuing the work at his own expense.

By then, Koch had become the director of the Institute for Infectious Diseases in Berlin, and, in 1890, he invited Ehrlich to work there. Ehrlich was only too happy to accept the opportunity of research in the distinguished laboratory. Here he began to work with Emil von Behring.

The excitement created by von Behring's discovery of diphtheria antitoxin was at its height. But the results in the clinic were disappointing. Von Behring's serum was too weak to do the job of protecting against diphtheria. For a time it looked as though the remedy was a complete failure. Ehrlich stepped in to help von Behring out of the difficulty.

Von Behring was unable to obtain a high potency of the diphtheria antitoxin, and Ehrlich pointed out to him the solution of the problem. He worked out a precise method of measuring the curative value of the antitoxin in definite units. As a result of being able to measure exactly the amount of antitoxin, it became possible, by repeated injections in ever increasing amounts, to produce a higher concentration of antitoxin units. The strength of the serum rose higher and higher until an effective potency was attained.

Both the method and the standards that Ehrlich established to determine the potency of the serum solved not only the problem of effectiveness of diphtheria antitoxin, but also became the accepted technique for measuring the protectiveness of sera in other diseases that are produced by toxins. Ehrlich's intervention made the diphtheria serum treatment practical and reliable.

The happy cooperation between Ehrlich and von Behring early in their careers came to a sad end, just when the time came to produce the serum on a large scale. A chemical firm interested in manufacturing it for medical use was supposed to have offered both of them a share in the profit from the discovery. The story surrounding the negotiations as told by Ehrlich's devoted and admiring secretary leaves no doubt that Ehrlich was deeply hurt and disillusioned.

When discussions of the terms of the contract were arranged, Ehrlich received a telegram to come immediately to the chemical works, where he was awaited by von Behring and a representative of the company. It seems that the plan von Behring had in mind was that Ehrlich would work as Director of a State Institute, then not yet in existence. Counting on his influence with the government authorities, von Behring would get Ehrlich appointed as director of such an institute. This would mean, of course, that as director he would not be permitted to receive money from a private chemical firm, and would have to be released from the contract.

Ehrlich, greatly excited at the thought of being free to do research according to his own ideas, paid little attention to the small print of the proposed contract. In the course of the conversation, the representative mentioned that it would not be possible for the firm to take on the financial burden of paying *both* investigators, a detail that escaped Ehrlich.

As it turned out, von Behring's influence was insufficient to keep his promise to help Ehrlich get the position at the Institute. So that ended Ehrlich's dream of a well-equipped laboratory where he could carry on his experiments according to his own plans. But von Behring established himself as the head of the Behring-Works in Marburg, from which he received an enormous income for the rest of his life. The incident which resulted in the estrangement of the two men was a source of life-long bitterness for Ehrlich.

How Ehrlich estimated his own contribution to their joint

work can be gleaned from a letter he wrote to a friend at the turn of the century.

"He . . . [Behring] seems to have had the idea that I should work for him for a small wage and help *him* to find new discoveries and make millions! He owes his success with the diphtheria serum, especially his big material success, to *me*. When we started to work together his serum contained only ¼ to ½ a unit of antitoxin per c.c., while mine had thirty. I had worked with ruminants, goats and cows, whereas he had used horses which give much stronger antitoxins. . . ."

Using horse serum and Ehrlich's method, von Behring was able to raise the units to 100 or more in each cubic centimeter. But later Ehrlich was able to get this yield even with goat serum.

The incident by which Ehrlich considered himself tricked might have been forgotten except for the fact that after Ehrlich had finally become the Director of the State Institute for Experimental Therapy in Frankfort, von Behring repeatedly sought his help in the making of new preparations. Ehrlich objected, explaining to the Prussian Ministry, that ". . . I do not think the Institute should undertake part of the preliminary experimental work to discover an effective preparation and so relieve the inventor of work which he should do himself." The demand for such work he said was unjustified, for the Institute "must remain independent and distinct from all private concerns . . ."

The refusal of the Ministry to honour von Behring's application for assistance did not improve his relations with Ehrlich whom he considered responsible for the rebuff.

While von Behring continued in his flourishing enterprise to develop new preparations against tetanus and tuberculosis in his magnificent "mountain laboratory," Ehrlich worked under very different conditions.

While in Koch's laboratory he was invited, in 1896, to become the director of a small State Institute for the Investigation and Control of Sera, in a suburb of Berlin. The government thus planned to establish controls over diphtheria serum and any others that would be found. The laboratory was an abandoned bakery; an old stable housed the animals. The budget was inadequate and, to clear up his deficits, Ehrlich had to make regular pleas for additional appropriations.

Ehrlich was not one to make himself unhappy over primitive laboratory conditions. When an occasional visitor remarked on the makeshift equipment, he would say cheerfully, "As long as I have a water tap, a flame, and some blotting paper, I can just as well work in a barn." Fritz, in a big blue apron served as his "animal nurse"; in a clean white overall, his hands washed and disinfected, he doubled as a laboratory assistant.

For three years Ehrlich worked like a demon, unsparing of his energies, following out every new idea of his imaginative mind. His work was fruitful, every publication containing some important contribution to science and medicine. To Ehrlich, the world owes the discovery that a toxin can be made much less toxic by changing it chemically to a toxoid—toxin-like but still capable of immunizing.

It was in this unimposing laboratory that he first conceived his theory of how the antibodies are formed and act in the blood. This was his memorable "side-chain" theory, the first attempt to explain how the body reacts to an invading organism. According to this theory the invader is the *antigen* which becomes attached to a *receptor,* a part of the defending substance, the *antibody,* which is always present in trace amounts.

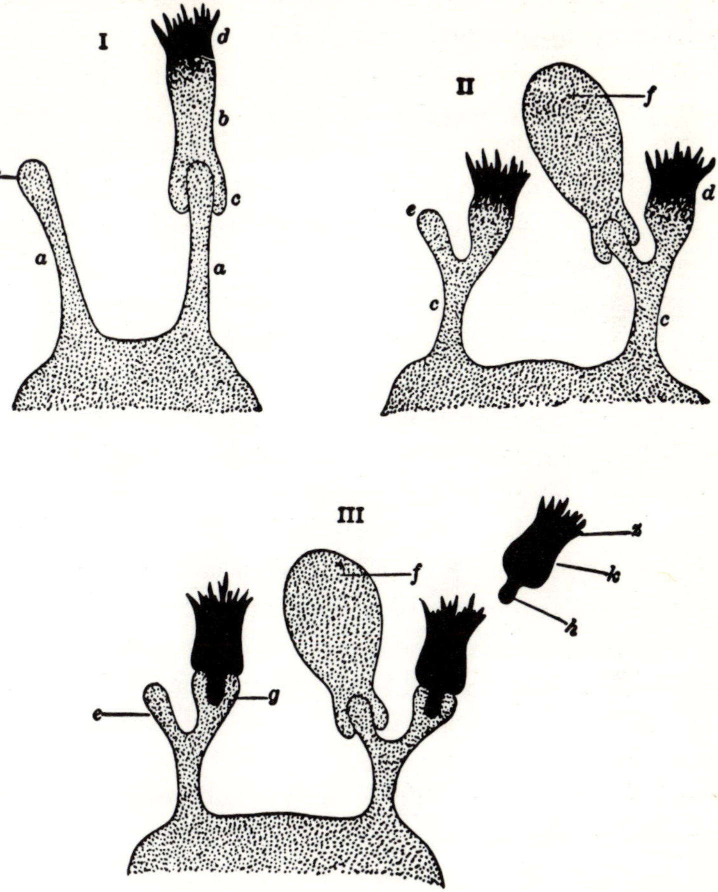

Ehrlich's diagram illustrating the side-chain theory: the hooking on of toxin to the antibody

Each antigen hooks on to a specific type of antibody, just as a key fits only a certain lock. When an antigen is injected in increasing amounts, the particular receptor regenerates at an increasing rate, hooking on to more of the antigen.

Much of this theory is no longer accepted, but it served as the basis for increasing the potency of diphtheria antitoxin by increasing repeated doses of toxin. "There must be mathematical laws which govern the way these toxins and antitoxins work," he once insisted to von Behring. His brilliant theory, though it was shown later to have many exceptions, worked: increasing the amount of toxin gradually increased the potency of the antitoxin.

Ehrlich was a creator of ideas, a genius who saw way ahead of other men, and of his time. The story is told of one time when he had moved to a large laboratory and was surrounded by dozens of assistants. Always under the scrutiny of government budget-makers, state institutes had to justify their expenditures. One day when an inspector came to see what was going on, he gathered the entire staff, and asked them: "But what does Herr Ehrlich do?" For a moment there was silence; then one assistant answered: "Why, Ehrlich thinks."

In 1899, a new and impressive laboratory was established in Frankfurt, The "Serum Institute," and Ehrlich became its director. Here he had two properly equipped working rooms, a room for cleaning glassware, a library, reading room, and a crew of able assistants. Kadereit, his faithful factotum, did everything from sharpening his pencils to keeping away unwanted visitors; Martha Marquardt, his tireless secretary, looked after the myriads of details in the life of the indefatigable little man who did the work of ten.

Ehrlich had a novel way of directing his own work as well as that of his assistants and collaborators. In the evening at home he would write the instructions for each worker on notecards he called "blocks." These were index cards of two sizes and various colours, each with serial numbers. Every morning Kadereit would bring the mail to Ehrlich's house; he opened it while he was taking his scanty breakfast. Then Kadereit would carry the mail along with the heap of "blocks" to the Institute, and place them on the working table of each of the men to whom they were addressed.

Back at the Institute, Kadereit would prepare what Ehrlich would need for his experiments, refill bottles with solutions and dyes, set up test tubes, sharpen his coloured pencils, file letters, send telegrams and, of course, make sure that there was a supply of his master's strong cigars, and a jug of mineral water. By then, Ehrlich usually arrived by horse-drawn cab, having read some manuscript or document on the way.

The master, or, as Kadereit called him, the "father," would leave his little dachshund in Kadereit's room, enter his study, a narrow room with only one unoccupied chair. The bookcase, shelves, desks, the sofa, and two other chairs were all put to but one use. They held books, manuscripts, reports, journals, and papers. New papers would always go on top. When a visitor was expected, the pile would be removed by Kadereit, to make one chair available. For a group of guests, the heap on the sofa was removed and placed underneath it, each piece undisturbed on the pile.

This accumulation over the years was not a whim of Ehrlich's or a sign of untidiness. He always knew where in the heap he had laid the particular book or periodical he wanted. Appearances mattered little to a man whose brain was perpetually buzzing with problems and plans for solving them.

A colleague wrote about Ehrlich after his death:

"Often very impatient during his daily work, Ehrlich would devote years of the most intensive work to solving a question to his satisfaction if this were at all possible. His laboratory work was free from all restrictions of orthodox procedure, so much so that he often gave orders which were quite contrary

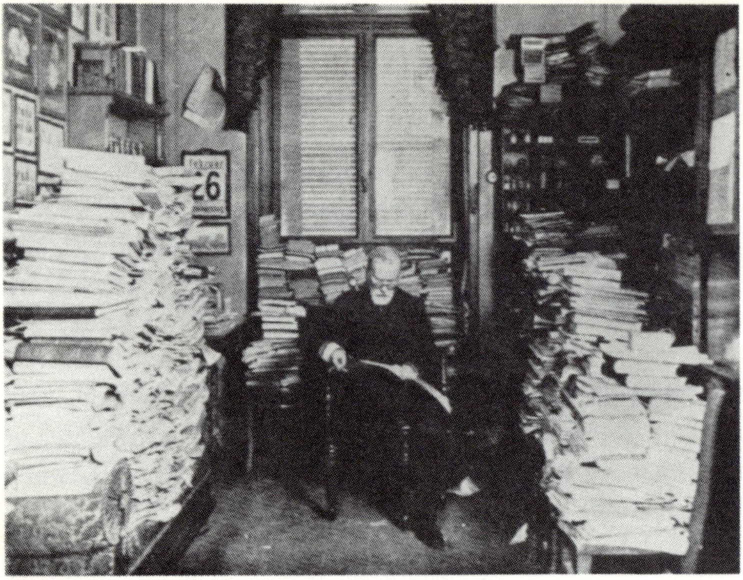

Dr. Paul Ehrlich in his famous study

to all rules and customs; but even the most extraordinary methods, when used in his experiments, would lead to the successful conclusions he expected. He was unaccustomed to going ahead slowly in one direction; and yet, in spite of this, even the most painstaking work could not ever quite satisfy his demand for precision."

For all his preoccupation with his work and impatience with careless errors he was the soul of kindness. Warmly generous whether with friends, colleagues, the maid who dropped his breakfast tray, or the laboratory porter who let the mice out of the jar, he endeared himself to the people around him.

Immersed in his own work to the point of apparently absent-minded exclusion of everything else, he never forgot the experiments he suggested to others or to inquire about the progress of their work. Sometimes a suggestion would go on one of his coloured "blocks": "It would perhaps be profitable if you would also take the vital dyeing with methylene blue into the field of your investigations," he wrote on a "block" to a British colleague.

Always ready to expound one of his theories even if the listener was not a scientist, he once tried to explain the "side-chain" idea to a visiting Berlin government representative.

When the listener seemed not to grasp his meaning, he said: "But this is very easy to demonstrate. I will make a drawing and show you. . . ." When the coloured pencil he held was blunt, he had another idea. Excusing himself for a moment he went into the laboratory, and returned with a piece of chalk.

"I shall draw it here," and he got on the floor to make his diagram.

The culmination of Ehrlich's remarkable career was in a field known today as chemotherapy, the treatment of disease with chemicals rather than with sera. In this work, Ehrlich was the groundbreaker of a path which led to the development of the modern "wonder drugs."

In Ehrlich's day only antitoxins were used to neutralize the toxins produced by invading germs. Ehrlich soon realized that only in certain diseases—diphtheria and tetanus—did the bacteria manufacture a poison which leaks out into the blood. These diseases could be cured by antitoxin, a way in which nature accomplishes the job. To imitate nature was logical. But diseases such as sleeping sickness, malaria, or syphilis could not be cured by antitoxic sera. Another method was necessary.

Ehrlich knew from his study with dyes that certain chemicals attach themselves to parts of the cell. From this he got the idea of using dyes and other chemical substances to hook on to an invading germ, but without hurting the tissues. Here was the first stumbling block—the chemical must not only work; it should also be harmless.

The marvellous effect of an antibody in a serum is that it anchors the parasites without damaging the body cells, he clearly saw. "The antibodies are Magic Bullets, which find their target by themselves. Hence their astonishingly specific effect, but with chemicals we can never count on such complete success and must concentrate all our powers on making the aim as accurate as we can contrive, so as to strike at the parasites as hard and the body cells as lightly as possible."

Then he and his growing group of students from far and wide went in search of man-made "Magic Bullets."

In 1904, with Dr. Shiga, a pupil of Kitasato in Tokyo, he began experiments on the trypanosome parasite which ravaged native Africans with sleeping sickness. They produced the disease in mice and then began the search of the right chemical. A large number of substances were tried without effect; the mice died as their blood was swarming with the parasites. Then they stumbled on a relative of a dye called trypan red which showed some action against the organisms. But it didn't dissolve easily in the blood. "Perhaps we can change it a little," he suggested to Shiga; "maybe then it will spread through the blood."

He rushed to his chemist friends in the nearby chemical works. Chemists had not yet advanced to the point where they could prepare chemicals to order. Some thought Ehrlich was slightly mad to think of such a thing. Others were loath to risk their reputation on what they thought was a scientific gamble. But Ehrlich persisted, and finally his dye was "changed a little" by the addition of one after another of different chemical groups. Then followed a long series of experiments to test the activity and the harmlessness of each in the animal. Finally, from a useless dye a cure was obtained. It both cured and prevented sleeping sickness in mice.

By this series of experiments, Ehrlich accomplished many "firsts."

It was the first cure of a disease produced in the laboratory.

For the first time the cure was a chemical substance created by man, synthesized in a laboratory.

Also, it was a chemical made to order, so the chemists knew its exact composition.

This was the beginning of a new era in the treatment of infections. But only the beginning. From then on, the methods worked out by Ehrlich, while constantly battling his sceptical chemists, would be applied to malaria, relapsing fever, other tropical diseases, and syphilis.

Then one day in 1905, the discovery of the spirochete organism which causes syphilis was announced at a Congress in Vienna. It was only a "preliminary report," but a year later when its discoverers were certain that they had bagged the killer, one of them came to visit Ehrlich. Since this organism was thought to resemble the trypanosomes, perhaps one of the many of Professor Ehrlich's preparations could be tried on their clinic patients.

Taking his visitor to the chemotherapy laboratory which had been set up for Ehrlich by a wealthy woman, he introduced him to his chemists who were working under his direction but without his conviction. He stopped to speak to one of them, explaining that to preserve the potency of the chemical they were preparing, they would have to exclude the oxygen. "Think over how this can best be done, and give me your report. This is absolutely necessary, Dr. Bertheim."

The next morning as usual Kadereit was delivering the "blocks" to each of the men. Dr. Bertheim looked at his, and immediately tore it up in anger. When Ehrlich arrived in the laboratory, he went to Bertheim's bench, to inquire what he had found out about the method of preparation. Scarcely looking up, Bertheim said:

"What method, Herr Professor?"

"What I told you yesterday—that the preparations must be protected by excluding oxygen."

"No," was the sullen reply.

"I have also written you a 'block' about it! Where is that 'block,' Dr. Bertheim?" Ehrlich now demanded angrily.

Finally interrupting his work, the chemist acknowledged that he had torn it up.

In a rage, Ehrlich ordered Kadereit immediately to bring the duplicate book, in which he always had a copy of each "block." Ehrlich raved and shouted, swinging his arms and hurling epithets at the stubborn fools who disregarded his directions.

"I do not give my directions for fun! If I give an order, it is urgently necessary! And I expect it to be carried out."

Pointing to the page with his directions, he shouted: "If my instructions are not attended to, if we do not protect our preparations by the absolute exclusion of oxygen and bottle them in a vacuum, deaths will occur, and the preparations will have to be thrown on the dung heap. . . . Please note the contents of the 'block' and let me know *this very day* what you propose to do!"

Resistance of this sort by men with much narrower vision than Ehrlich's often delayed the work—work that involved long series of trials with animals, repeated over and over again for months. Hundreds of compounds had to be discarded, others tried with meticulous care over years of patient labour.

In 1909, Kitasato sent another pupil to study with the world-renowned, Nobel-Prize-winning Ehrlich. Hata, just ar-

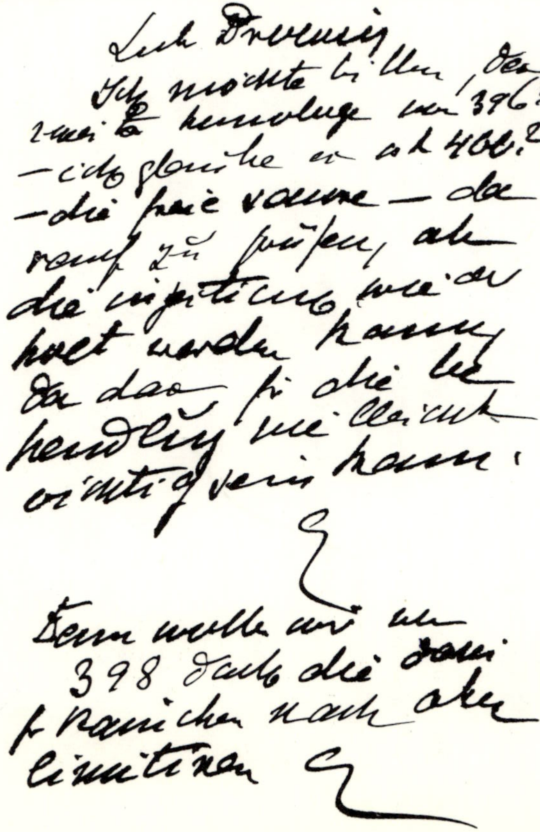

Lieb Browning
Ich möchte bitten, den
zweiten homologen von 396?
— ich glaube es ist 400? —
— die freie Säure — da-
rauf zu prüfen, ob
die injection wieder-
holt werden kann
da das für die Be-
handlung vielleicht
wichtig sein kann.
E

Dann wollen wir an
398 doch die Dosis
f. Kaninchen nach oben
limitieren E

TRANSLATION

I would like to request that you test the second homolog of 396 (?)—I think it is 400 (?)—the free acid—to see if the injection can be repeated because this might be important for the treatment.

E [Ehrlich]

Then we want to limit the highest dose of 398 for rabbits after all.

E [Ehrlich]

One of Ehrlich's "blocks": a note written by him, advising C. H. Browning, now Professor of Tropical Medicine, on the work for the next day rived from Tokyo, had found a way to produce syphilis in rabbits.

"Professor Kitasato tells me you have great skill in inoculating rabbits with this disease, Dr. Hata. I would like you to continue with the work here." To which Dr. Hata politely bowed.

"Very happy, Herr Professor," he said radiantly and went to work, trying different compounds on his sick rabbits.

Among the hundreds of compounds two—No. 418 and No. 606—seemed to Ehrlich to show the greatest promise. But one of the workers to whom Ehrlich gave No. 606 to try out reported no results and it was laid aside as worthless.

While doctors were treating patients with No. 418, Hata found that No. 606 which, because of the doubting chemists, had been set aside, was actually better.

"I believe 606 is *very* efficacious," the Japanese doctor announced one day to the excited Ehrlich.

Pacing up and down the laboratory, Ehrlich was talking to himself: "I always had a strong feeling—have been convinced for two years—that 606 *must be good!* . . . But Dr. R., the incapable *good-for-nothing,* saw nothing."

And it *was* good. Salvarsan—606—arsphenamine, by whatever name it went, this arsenic compound showed itself to be the cure in the human test that followed.

In 1954, one hundred years after Ehrlich was born, third-generation disciples of his in the United States arranged a Paul Ehrlich Centennial. Two bronze portrait busts of Emil von Behring and Paul Ehrlich (born a day apart) were presented to the New York Academy of Sciences. His Excellency Heinz L. Krekeler, Ambassador of the Federal Republic of

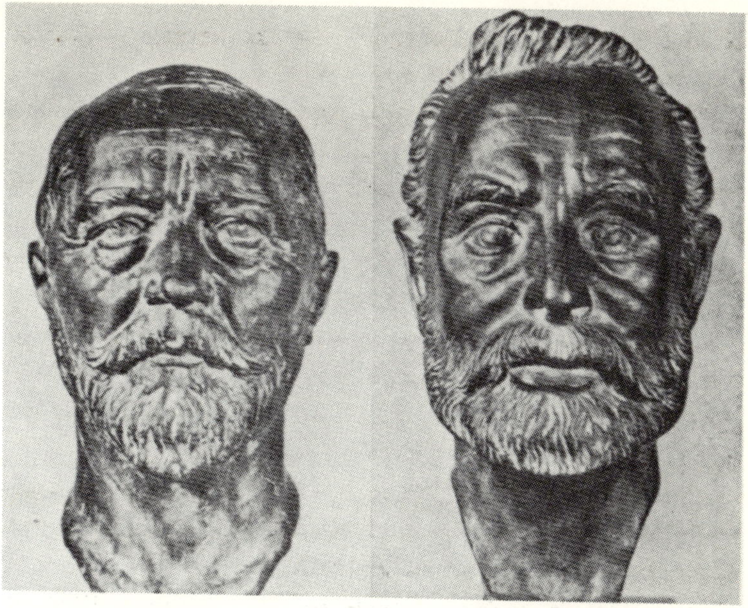

Busts of von Behring and Ehrlich presented to the New York Academy of Sciences in 1954

Germany, presented them on behalf of the Farbewerke Hoechst, in Frankfort, a dye and chemical firm that helped in the discoveries. On this occasion, a number of scientists, each a specialist in a field in which Ehrlich had pioneered, discussed the work Ehrlich had done in that field: his influence on chemistry, his contributions to the knowledge of immunity, to the cancer problem, the conquest of trypanosomes, spirochetes, his work on vital staining, on the intimate structure of blood cells, in chemotherapy and the resistance of bacteria to drugs.

A century ago the genius of Paul Ehrlich charted the way for scientists in many fields, and still illumines the path to more discoveries.

9

DIPHTHERIA CONQUERED

Béla Schick (1877–)

On July 16, 1877 a baby boy was born in his granduncle's home in the little Hungarian town of Boglar on Lake Balaton. The baby's brother and their mother Janka (Johanna Schick) were visiting her uncle, Dr. Sigismund Telegdy, when Béla arrived prematurely. What made his mother take the long trip of eighty or more miles from their home in Graz, southeastern Austria, is hard to tell. Perhaps it was foolhardy in her condition, but it turned out well in the end. Luckily, Dr. Telegdy was there to deliver the premature infant, despite the complications of a difficult birth.

The Schick baby, weighing hardly more than three pounds, had a slim chance to survive, except for his uncle's fond and expert care. It was only right that he should pick the name of Béla (pronounced Bayla) which is Hungarian, and didn't go with Béla's Austrian last name. Uncle Sigismund felt he had the right to exact another tribute from his favourite niece. When Janka was well enough to listen, he sat on the edge of her bed with an air of having something important to say.

"Janka, the Lord has blessed you with two sons, but I feel that Béla is at least half mine; I saved him."

Janka opened her large blue eyes even wider, wondering what her uncle was going to ask of her now.

"Let Jacob decide what he wants Richard to be—a merchant, an engineer, or even a philosopher—but Béla must be a doctor."

He paused, probably startled by his own words, for Richard was hardly out of his first year, and Béla was still not as big as a normal newborn baby. But after a moment he continued as if the matter had been settled.

"Perhaps he may even become a great doctor, and save many lives."

When it was safe enough for Frau Schick to travel, she returned home with her two babies, where their father anxiously awaited them. If she had given any thought at all to her uncle's plans for Béla, she was too busy with the bustle of life at home and the care of two young children to bother to discuss with Jacob a possibility that was so far in the future. But the wise and learned doctor in Boglar never gave up his dream for his nephew's life work. In fact, it became a passion with him as he watched the boy grow up.

Béla remembered the many childhood visits to Uncle Sigismund's home. When he was old enough to travel alone, it was even more fun because then he and his uncle could spend many hours talking as "man to man." It was a great big wonderful secret that Béla shared with his uncle. Uncle Sigismund was a rare healer and his patients adored the country doctor. But for Béla there was the wonder and mystery surrounding the stories his uncle told about the history of medicine. Through them he was transported into the world of great discoveries, of trailblazing adventures by brave and deeply curious men who sought answers to perplexing questions.

Béla spent part of his summer vacations with Uncle Sigismund. In the evening, when the doctor had sent his last patient home, he would take the boy with him on his accustomed walk along the lake.

"Béla, would you believe that two thousand years ago people thought that food was turned into something called 'natural spirits' in the liver?" his uncle once asked without expecting an answer.

"And do you know that they once thought that a lapis stone would stop bad nose bleeds, and that ashes of the stork would protect them against poisons and pests?"

But even in those days there were thoughtful men who didn't believe in spirits, magic, or charms, his uncle explained on another occasion. Then he went on to tell about Herophilus, in ancient Alexandria, who dissected human corpses and found that the arteries were filled, not with air, but with blood. And 500 years before Christ, the Greek doctor Alcmaeon had examined the bodies of animals and had seen that the brain governed their movements. Even before that, the Egyptians learned how to embalm corpses, and in India and China surgeons performed delicate operations with great skill, even though they had no anesthetics; and they also learned to extract hundreds of curative drugs from herbs.

Always brave men had to defy superstition and taboos to get at the truth; to get answers that made sense. It took courage to fight beliefs in evil spirits, and in the power of magic and angry gods. The courageous and obstinate wanted to know what caused disease, and above all, they aimed to learn how to heal the sick. The followers of the great Hippocrates, Dr. Telegdy told Béla, took the solemn oath: "In all my treatment I will strive so far as lies in my power for the benefit of the patients . . ."

"Don't ever forget that, Béla, when you get to be a doctor yourself." How could he, as he lay awake that night, deter-

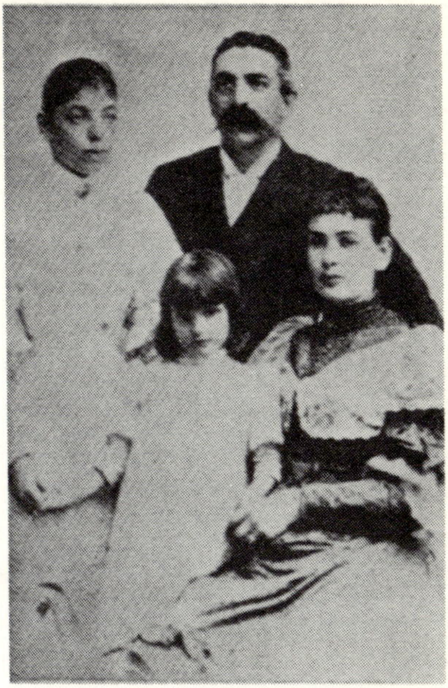

Béla Schick's parents and sisters

mined that he, too, would be one of those "obstinate" men? As much as young Béla wished to keep his big secret to himself, his parents couldn't help discovering that with each visit to Boglar, the boy picked up a kind of grown-up wisdom.

By the time Béla had finished the four-year local school, and followed his brother to the Staats Gymnasium in Graz, he had two little sisters—Frieda born when he was eleven, and Ilona several years later. But schoolboys approaching their teens have little interest in baby sisters, except perhaps to tease them. In the happy Schick household the two boys got along as scrappingly as in most families. Richard early showed a talent for music, and his father saw to it that there was a piano in the house, making sure that the boy would work hard at it. While young Béla was dreaming of being a doctor like his hero uncle, he also liked to play the piano, and of course, always just at the time when Richard was practising. And so there was boyish screaming, kicking, and fighting, until the family thought of a way out.

Béla loved animals and so Papa Schick brought home a big Newfoundland dog for Béla's very own. Immersed in Roman history, Béla named him Caesar, who unlike his namesake was friendly, obedient, and devoted to his master. For a time Béla gloried in the companionship of the dog, taking him for walks in the woods, and for long swims in the nearby river. Richard soon felt he had the worst of the bargain. In exchange for the chance to romp with Caesar, he let Béla play the piano now and then. Béla became interested enough to take lessons and it wasn't long before the Schick boys were playing duets and even writing their own music, while Caesar patiently listened until it was time to run around with the boys.

But one day this blissful trio met with tragedy. After one of those long swims, Caesar became sick, and the boys tried to nurse him back to health in the woodshed. When he was getting no better, Béla's alarm sent him running for the veterinarian. By then it was too late, and the next morning Caesar was dead. Even more than the loss of his cherished friend was the distressing thought that he didn't know the cause of the dog's death. It must have been Uncle Sigismund who whispered to him across many miles from Boglar. He would perform an autopsy, and find out.

Armed with the sharpest kitchen knife, he shut himself up in the shed thinking that Caesar's death was his own secret, not knowing that the vet had told his parents of his visit. Just as he was about to undertake his post-mortem, the door swung open, and there stood horrified Janka and Jacob.

Perhaps memories of his own youth made Jacob Schick take

pause before saying flatly "No." Somehow he understood the boy's feelings, that he just couldn't bury the dog before learning how he died. In fact, Béla himself had a solution which saved everybody's face. He would help the doctor perform the operation. That afternoon the veterinarian returned, and with Béla's assistance performed an autopsy. No, Caesar had not died from pneumonia, but from natural causes—old age.

At eighteen Béla was a young man with considerable knowledge, a graduate of the Staats Gymnasium where he had received a good education in the classics, languages, mathematics, and science. A serious student, he had done his work to the satisfaction of his teachers and to the amazement of his fellow students. Why, they wondered, would Béla prefer to spend his time in the library rather than at play? His required homework over, Béla searched out every book he could find on biology, natural sciences, and the history of science. His absorption in these subjects came from his secret ambition to become a doctor like his Uncle Sigismund.

But Jacob Schick had a different career in mind for his son. Herr Schick was a grain merchant, and planned to have both his sons join him in the granary. Together they would expand the business and become prosperous, and when he died his sons would carry on a well-established firm. Jacob Schick was thinking only of what seemed to him best for his boys. He was a devoted father and wished to see them have a comfortable life and perhaps build up a fortune greater than he had been able to achieve. This is not to say that he put money above other things. After all he did see to it that his children were educated in the best manner of the time. He would not be ashamed of them in the best company. They could hold their own even in a philosophical discussion. Not every merchant's son had a Gymnasium education, read Latin and French as well as German, studied music, and took dancing lessons.

It could never be said that Jacob Schick had no appreciation of the cultural things of life. He himself had dreamed, valued the arts, read books, studied history, and conversed intelligently on politics.

It never occurred to Papa Schick that Béla would have his own ideas of a future. In all other matters Jacob Schick was master in his household, and his children would not have thought of disobeying him. They had been brought up in strict discipline, and never questioned his right to make decisions for them. Janka also dutifully accepted her husband's wishes as law and found it best to avoid disagreements.

When Béla decided to follow not in his father's but in his uncle's footsteps there was bound to be a showdown, because both father and son were obstinate. Jacob could see only the long, hard years ahead in the study of medicine. In fact, he reminded Janka, at Béla's age, he himself had had ideas of becoming a doctor but had finally turned to the greater security of a grain merchant. And his sons would have the advantage of an established business, he told Janka.

Jacob considered a Gymnasium education enough, but not Béla. His extensive reading had only whetted his appetite for further study. Should he become a merchant or go on to study medicine? Upon graduation in 1895 Béla decided it was time to convince his father that he knew his own mind where his career was concerned.

One evening he approached his father with the earnestness of a youth who has learned a great deal more than his school assignments demanded. Béla was familiar not only with the history of past contributions in medicine, but he also knew of the work then going on in European laboratories. In France,

Louis Pasteur had inspired a great many scientists to work in the new and exciting field of bacteriology. Béla had read of their achievements, just as today some young people read everything in sight on their favourite subjects of photography, electronics, or rockets. He began by telling his father of some brand new experiments. Jacob Schick knew that his son was serious, for a boy of his age, and his knowledge impressed him. Scientists in Germany and France were working in a newly discovered world of life, Béla related. They were studying diseases that couldn't be cured with the old familiar drugs, diseases caused by a strange, different kind of enemy—microbes. Although too small to see without a microscope, they were deadly once they got a foothold in the body.

Béla told how Edwin Klebs had actually seen one of these microbes—the diphtheria bacillus—under his microscope, and how Loeffler had grown it in pure culture in test tubes, learned about its "habits," and by injecting it into animals had given them the disease. The scientist had also found thriving "Klebs-Loeffler" bacilli in the throat of every child who was suffering from diphtheria.

Béla was now talking about his favourite subject. For centuries diphtheria had been a terrifying children's disease. As long ago as the sixth century a Mesopotamian doctor had told about the "croup" that choked its little victims to death. Then in 1826, Pierre Bretonneau of Tours, France gave it its modern name and described its symptoms—fever, flushed face, dry throat, painful, gasping breathing, and finally suffocation. Without the knowledge about germs people were helpless against it.

Béla went on with the story: the first step in the conquest of a bacterial disease had now been accomplished. There was no doubt that a bacillus was causing the disease. Meanwhile, in Pasteur's laboratory in Paris, Emil Roux and Alexandre Yersin had discovered the toxin produced in the tissues by the bacillus. Even without the presence of bacteria, the toxin, when injected alone, gave animals the disease.

Next Béla told about von Behring and Kitasato, the scientists who discovered immune substances in the blood serum of animals infected with diphtheria. In the same way, Kitasato had earlier found a serum for tetanus, Béla explained. This discovery, which was only three years old, had not yet been printed in Béla's textbooks, but he had read all the medical reports in the library.

The work of von Behring and Kitasato had raised high hopes for a diphtheria antitoxin, but the results were at first disappointing: the antitoxin was too weak to be a cure. Then Paul Ehrlich had joined von Behring in the Institute for Infectious Disease in Berlin, Béla went on. There, under Robert Koch, its director, they had worked out a way to produce large amounts of antitoxin. By repeated injections with diphtheria toxin they produced it in the blood of horses. This horse serum had enough antibodies to neutralize the toxin and cure animals sick with diphtheria. Also, with a method devised by Ehrlich, its potency could be measured—so many *units* of diphtheria-fighting strength.

Béla Schick had followed these developments closely, not out of idle curiosity, but because of his consuming desire to join in the work. So why couldn't he become a medical scientist and help to make such discoveries? Perhaps a way could be found to *prevent* the disease!

Herr Schick's business activities had pushed into the background his own student days when he had read about medicine and ancient doctors. He had been fascinated by the contributions of Hippocrates, the father of medicine. In those days doctors had no instruments for examining patients, no thermometers, no listening tubes, no way of measuring the force of blood against the walls of the vessels. But Hippocrates had a wonderful eye for seeing just what was necessary to find out what ailed the patient. And then there were his Aphorisms —great sayings that stood the test of centuries: "One man's meat is another man's poison." "Desperate diseases need desperate remedies." There was a great man! Herr Schick was caught up in Béla's enthusiastic recital of stirring medical discoveries, and these touched off his own lively imagination. He was also wise enough to recognize that his son's ambition was no passing fancy.

No, Béla was not one of those idle drifters who aimlessly pursued one course after another in a university, never "making anything of themselves." One by one Jacob's objections to a university career for his son faded, as he became convinced that Béla was ready to undertake the hard work and the many sacrifices his goal would demand. His father would no longer stand in his way! That autumn, 1895, Béla Schick entered as a medical student in the Karl Franz University of Graz.

"Before you learn to walk you must learn to crawl," Uncle Sigismund often repeated. Just so, Béla Schick had to learn a great deal before he could begin research on his own, for there was a long road between reading about the work of other scientists and taking up where they had left off.

How right was dear old Uncle Sigismund! One must not only study books, but observe, practice, and heal before going on to research. Like Thomas Sydenham, the great English physician of two centuries earlier, he would say: "You must go to the bedside. It is there alone you can learn disease." Béla was grateful to Uncle Sigismund for letting him work at the bedside when he visited his Boglar patients with him.

Was Béla just lucky in having an outstanding professor who started him on the road he wanted to travel, or was it a case of the professor recognizing a promising student? Whichever was the case, when thoughtful and earnest Béla came under the influence of the brilliantly stimulating young Professor Kraus he was bound to make long strides. Professor Kraus chose him to assist with demonstrations and initiated him into the exciting work of laboratory experimentation. Three mornings a week he helped the Professor arrange demonstrations of puzzling cases for the students to diagnose. Diagnosis was no guesswork. First you had to observe, get the facts and yet more facts. In animals you could study other facts, experiment, obtain knowledge that made diagnosis a science.

In his courses on the diseases of the nervous system, Béla became immersed in the mysteries of the disordered brain. When, under Professor Escherich who had been brought up in the new school of bacteriologists (he had himself discovered the bacillus that bears his name and that lives harmlessly in the human intestine), he learned to look in the hidden world of microbes for the cause of disease.

All this was bound to steer him away from the plans his mother and uncle had for him, when he should become a doctor. She hoped Béla would marry and raise a family, and he that Béla would take his place at Boglar, and become a doctor popular with the fashionable folk who came for water cures to the lovely shores of Lake Balaton. Janka made no headway with resolute Béla. As for Uncle Sigismund, Janka would just put him off with letters that kept him wondering and hoping.

Then one summer evening when Béla had only the last year of his medical studies to complete, the family was gathered to celebrate his twenty-second birthday. Uncle Sigismund took the long trip to be present on this important occasion which was more than just a birthday—it was so near the time when he would realize his dream of his nephew's future. Janka was supervising the preparations of the festive meal. Frieda was helping to set the table and little Ilona was getting under everybody's feet. Richard tried his best to go about his business as though it were just another day. Jacob noisily acted the man of the house, bubbling with pride: one son was about to become a doctor; the other was exhibiting his talents at the piano. Meanwhile Richard was doing his best to drown out the noise of the household with a composition by Richard Wagner, while Dr. Telegdy was feasting his eyes on the happy family scene and giving his quiet, warm approval. Only Béla had not yet arrived.

What was keeping him? It could be a number of things. Perhaps he was poring over some report in the library, forgetting the time, or an interesting case had kept him at the hospital. Janka hopefully thought it might even be a young lady. After all, it was time Béla interested himself in girls. And there were signs, she thought, that he was thinking of such things. He brushed his clothes neatly every morning, polished his shoes, nursed his newly grown little mustache and paid some attention to the mirror. As if to assure the others, but more herself Janka said: "He will be coming in any minute now."

Finally, the guest of honour arrived, not a little embarrassed for having kept everyone waiting. He was obviously in a state of tense excitement, but he had no simple explanation for his tardiness—such as having met someone in the street, or having overlooked the hour. It was Janka who spoke first, with an announcement that the steaming soup and roasted goose had just been set on the table, and that everyone had better take their seats. Only after they were part way through the dinner, Béla explained that he had been detained at the home of Professor Escherich.

Theodor Escherich, the head of Pediatrics, the department devoted to children's diseases, had invited him to meet Dr. Meinhard von Pfaundler, a new professor who would add lustre to the already famous children's clinic. In Béla, the inquisitive student, Professor Escherich recognized one who had the curiosity to travel on yet uncharted paths. Here was a young man who could apply the new knowledge of bacteriology to children's diseases. From Professor Kraus, Béla had learned to use the methods of science in medicine to combine laboratory experiments in animals with observation of patients in the clinic.

Béla must study in his department, Professor Escherich had proposed, in a way which implied that hardly any other course could be considered. The field of pediatrics was wide open. So few were working in the study of children's diseases. After completion of his medical course, he was to work closely with von Pfaundler for several more semesters, attend his lectures and clinics, and join him in his laboratory studies. Perhaps his professor had done him a good turn in steering him back to his early intentions to find a cure for diphtheria.

Béla was so engrossed in the telling of his story that he failed to notice that his family was stunned. So it wasn't, after all, some fine young lady with whom her son was planning to settle down! Marriage was furthest from his mind, Janka sadly thought. As to Jacob, the worst of his fears of an impractical future among dusty books, test tubes, and scientific papers was coming true. Béla was going to follow the path of a penniless scholar. But what could be done? Could he cut off his ambitious son without any financial help? Even if he could, would this make any difference in Béla's plans? Janka wouldn't let him think of such a thing. What was Dr. Telegdy thinking? He had been the one to encourage his nephew to take up medicine, had been his childhood inspiration. And now someone else would have to fill his shoes when the time came —when he would be called away from his patients forever. How was he going to take the blow, Janka wondered as she eyed her uncle anxiously? It was some time before Uncle Sigismund spoke: "On the occasion of your birthday and of your decision not to be a country doctor but a scientist, I extend to you my heartfelt wishes." And should Béla have any doubt of his uncle's sincerity, he added: "Should you ever need help, Béla, remember you can always count on me." Not forgetting the birthday, Dr. Telegdy took out the present he had brought —a watch on a heavy gold chain.

Béla was deeply stirred. He had expected opposition, but through his selfless, sincere gesture, the old doctor had helped the family accept Béla's plans. Richard too, felt the solemnity of the occasion. Yes, his brother was smarter than he. In the small town of Graz, word had spread that Béla was a promising student. He might yet make a name for himself, and bring honour to his family, Richard added.

Smiling Béla, pleased with the way things turned out, answered with quiet modesty: "I don't know whether you will have occasion to be proud of me, but of one thing I am sure—pediatrics is my life."

During the years that followed, Béla Schick completed his schooling, joined a clinic in a children's hospital, worked in the laboratory of an experimental institute in Vienna, soldiered in the army under his country's compulsory military service law, and finally returned to a modest hospital post to do research.

All this time Dr. Schick was living like the penniless scholar his father had envisioned. As long as he wasn't earning money Herr Schick sent him a monthly allowance of fifty kronen, one-fourth of which went to pay the rent for a tiny room with an iron bedstead, straw mattress, table, and chair. The hospital posts he held early in his career as researcher paid hardly more than his former allowance. But he gave no thought to money other than to keep himself alive, and when his uncle sent him an occasional sum, he bought a little extra food which Béla said helped him to work harder.

While working mainly in his favourite field, pediatrics, Dr. Schick never let up in his studies. He closely observed his child patients as he treated them, tried new remedies, experimented, made notes, wrote reports, and gave lectures in the clinic, for he was a professor as well as a doctor. He had already done important research in tuberculosis, scarlet fever, allergies, and children's diseases. But he must go on experimenting: there was always so much more to learn.

He was so involved in so many different experiments, that it is not surprising that his winding path of study and work brought him back to his youthful interest in diphtheria. Actually, his interest had never waned, for children were still dying all over the world during diphtheria epidemics. But now that he was a Professor in the Children's Clinic in Vienna he could concentrate on it, and did. Not only did Dr. Schick teach medical students but also he had children as his own patients, and was able to study them and to conduct experiments in the laboratory.

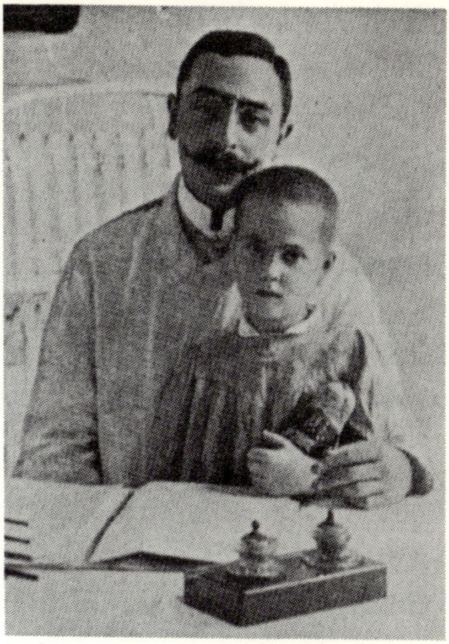

Béla Schick, in Vienna, in 1904, in scarlet fever ward of children's hospital

He made extensive studies of the antitoxin in human serum, and found that people who had recovered from diphtheria retained antibodies in their serum *throughout their lifetime,* and also that other people had them even though they didn't remember ever having had the disease! Eighty-five out of every hundred adults had these antibodies, which explained why grown-ups rarely contracted diphtheria. On the other hand, newborn infants were protected by antibodies acquired from their mothers during pregnancy or nursing.

But Dr. Schick also found that babies soon lost their early protection, and between the ages of one and five, most easily became victims of diphtheria. The first problem to solve was to find a test by which to discover who was and who wasn't protected. If he could do this, it would be possible to prevent the disease in those who were susceptible, and at the same time avoid the risk of sickness from the serum itself in those who were immune and needed no added protection.

He had already determined the amount of diphtheria antitoxin in human serum, and in the serum of children who had diphtheria. Working first with guinea pigs and then with children he discovered that a very small amount of toxin injected into the skin produced a reaction in some, and not in others. A minimal amount of the poison caused the skin to redden and swell at the spot where the toxin was injected. In these children, the amount of diphtheria antitoxin was low. In persons who did not show this reaction, he found that the serum contained enough of the protective antibodies to ward off the disease.

Here was an easy way of telling whether the serum of the child contained antitoxin, whether he would be immune to an attack of the disease, or if in the absence of antitoxin he might contract it.

In 1913 Dr. Schick was ready to announce to the world that he had been successful! In a brief but important article in a German medical weekly, he described the test which bears his name. In his own words translated from the German, Dr. Schick said in part:

A Skin Reaction with Diphtheria Toxin in Human Beings

For this injection the most important part is the needle, which must be very thin and its point very short, so that it reaches only the uppermost layers of the skin. The amount of injection is a tenth of a cubic centimeter [a tiny drop] and its strength is equal to 1/50 of the dose deadly to a 250-gram guinea pig. If the injection is done right, a white circle appears where the puncture is made. After eight hours, a red spot less than a half-inch appears, getting redder until it is brightest 48 hours after the injection. Then the skin over the spot blisters and shrivels, finally drying and peeling.

If no reaction develops at the place of injection it means immunity against the disease. This is called a *negative* reaction and proves the presence of those substances which neutralize the diphtheria toxin. If these substances are lacking, the red patch indicates a positive reaction. This means that the person is susceptible to diphtheria.

Perhaps you remember that although you had received a toxin shot when you were a baby, five years later the doctor found that you were not fully protected. Your *positive* Schick test meant that you needed a "booster" shot—more of the same toxin—to stimulate your body to manufacture more antitoxin, enough to keep you immune. If your reaction had been *negative,* the "booster" would have been unnecessary.

The importance of the Schick test is that it makes possible the separation of two classes of children: those who are protected and those who are not. The susceptible ones can be fully protected against diphtheria by a dose of diphtheria toxin. It is a small-scale sample of what would happen to a susceptible child if the bacilli invaded his throat tissues, grew there, and produced enormous amounts of toxin which spread through the entire bloodstream. Of course, antibodies would be formed, but not enough to neutralize the toxin. However, by injecting a small, *measured,* bit of toxin, the same reaction is much milder and safe. At the same time, it causes the body to make enough antitoxin to ward off a full-scale attack of diphtheria!

Wonderful as were the discoveries of diphtheria's cause, cure, and susceptibility test, they could not by themselves prevent epidemics. There still remained the enormous job of convincing people that their children could be made safe—a job that took a long, long time to accomplish.

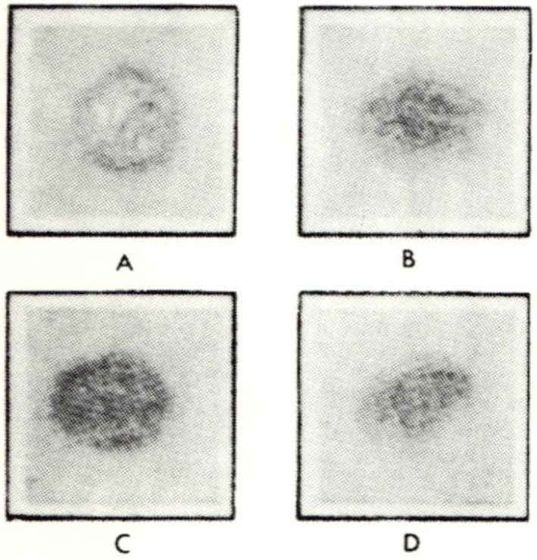

AFTER 48 HOURS

All grades of positive Schick reactions: A, B, C, D, from the most to the least positive. Patient A has practically no antitoxin, and is most susceptible, while D has some protection.

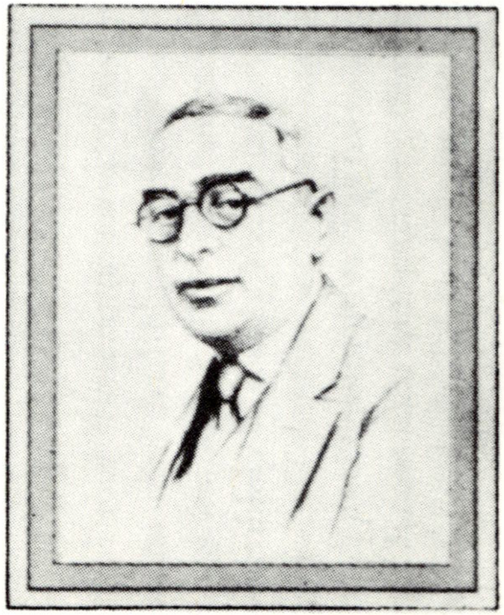

BÉLA SCHICK

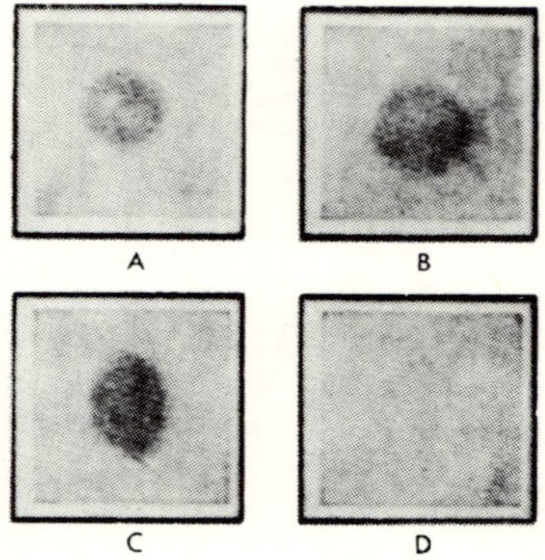

The reaction has faded: A is still red and scaling (1 week); B and C pigmentation of darkening is showing (2 and 3 weeks); D pigmentation is almost gone.

NO CHILD NEED HAVE DIPHTHERIA

Chart showing reactions to Schick test for diphtheria

Fourteen years after the Schick test was announced, there were still about 100,000 cases and 10,000 deaths from diphtheria in the United States. In New York City alone, 15,000 cases and 700 deaths were regularly reported each year until finally—as in other cities too—the New York Department of Health decided to enter the battle. Public campaigns were organized against the disease, with Diphtheria Prevention Committees planning the attack, just as an army's general staff does in wartime. Clinics were established to immunize children, and most important, a drive was started to educate *parents.*

What better way to reach the parents than through their children? A large insurance company and the Milbank Memorial Fund flooded the schools with millions of pieces of literature. "Train Tickets to No-Diphtheria Town," one was called; "To the Schick Test," was another. One contained the story of a little boy who had died of diphtheria. In large letters, the story began:

> YOUR CHILD NEED NOT HAVE DIPHTHERIA.
>
> Science has made it possible for you to give absolute protection to your child. Some children are protected by nature and will never contract the disease. Other children are susceptible to it. By means of the Schick Test you can find out to which class your child belongs . . .
>
> Children who might contract diphtheria as shown by the Schick Test may be protected against it by the Toxin-Antitoxin treatment . . .
>
> EVERY CHILD SHOULD BE SCHICK TESTED.
>
> YOU OWE IT TO YOUR CHILD.

Along with the pamphlet children brought home slips to be signed by their parents giving permission to test and immunize their children. Children who were tested wore large

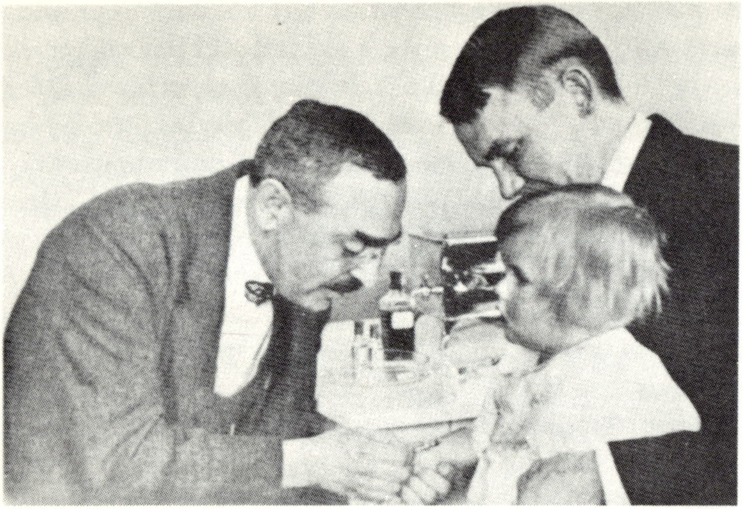

Dr. Schick performing the Schick test on a child

buttons, as if they were campaigning for a candidate for governor: "I AM SCHICKED: ARE YOU?"

Squarely in the centre of this critical battle stood Dr. Béla Schick, for in 1923 he had been invited to the United States to join the staff of one of New York's most famous hospitals. By 1927 he was the head of the city's Diphtheria Commission. One of his tasks was to persuade parents, because before granting permission for their children to be given the Schick test and immunization treatment, parents demanded to know: Are they really safe?

Quiet, modest Dr. Schick temporarily set aside his beloved work with children at the clinic to take on the greater job of saving millions. He lectured, wrote newspaper ads, and was persuaded to make radio addresses. On March 22, 1929, he broadcast this message:

> . . . 10,000 people died in the United States during 1927 from a disease which could have been avoided. What an amount of suffering, what an amount of sorrow could have been spared the parents of these children had they known this disease could have been avoided. . . .
>
> We know the germ which causes the disease, and we know that the germ, the diphtheria bacillus, produces a poison . . . diphtheria toxin, which endangers the health and the life of the child . . .
>
> Forty-eight special diphtheria prevention clinics are now being maintained by the Health Department, and . . . about 12,000 children have been completely immunized against the disease in these clinics. . . . I think parents who know that it is now possible to prevent diphtheria, and who nevertheless fail to have their children immunized, take a great responsibility upon their shoulders.

Dr. Schick had no children of his own, so he was unable to demonstrate personally his complete confidence in his work, as did Dr. Jonas Salk nearly thirty years later. But he persuaded his friend and co-worker, Dr. Abraham Zingher, to protect his children, and soon, one after another, doctors everywhere answered doubts and questions by immunizing their own children. And so gradually, if slowly, more and more parents lost their fears.

More and more children, shown by the Schick test to be susceptible to diphtheria, were given the toxin-antitoxin treatment—an injection of a mixture of both toxin and antitoxin—each week for three weeks.

Throughout the country the campaign went on, and everywhere with success. As soon as a child showed the first signs of diphtheria, antitoxin was given; this borrowed antitoxin helped him fight the disease until his own tissues began to make antibodies. Brothers, sisters, and other children who played with the patient were also injected. This protection with antitoxin didn't last, but it was good until the immediate danger was over. Then the children were given the three toxin-antitoxin injections and from then on they were immune to future infection.

In 1933 Dr. Schick was presented with an album containing the signatures of one million grateful New York children!

The laboratory struggle is long over. Methods have been perfected to measure the strength of toxin and antitoxin. A way has been found to make the toxin easier to take: it is first treated with formaldehyde, a chemical that changes it into *toxoid,* fully as effective, but producing no ill effects.

This is what your "booster" shot was. It took only a second and hurt no more than a pin prick. You didn't have to worry about the injection—the amount was so small it couldn't possibly make you sick. And by the time the doctor had finished telling you how it's done, he had already finished, and you hadn't even noticed it! In fact, you couldn't see the spot where the needle had penetrated your arm.

10

SCARLET FEVER NEXT

George F. and Gladys H. Dick (1881–   )

About the time when Béla Schick announced his skin test for diphtheria, an American-born doctor began to investigate the cause of scarlet fever. In 1912 when Dr. George F. Dick took up the study of this fever, which begins with a sore throat, develops into a skin rash, and ends with scaling and peeling a few weeks later, there were only guesses about its cause. "None of Koch's requirements had been met in its explanation," Dr. Dick wrote when his job was over a dozen or so years later.

The disease had been described some two-and-a-half centuries earlier by Sydenham, who gave it its name. The story of the discovery of its cause, prevention, and cure is a tale of careful and ingenious medical detective work—the "detectives," a man-and-wife team.

George Frederick Dick was born in Fort Wayne, Indiana in 1881. At the turn of the century he enrolled in Rush Medical School, University of Chicago, and after graduation interned at Cook County, one of the better known of Chicago's hospitals. He set up in practice in the town of Buhl, in the iron mining district of western Minnesota. In the first decade of the century, that was rugged frontier country where a doctor could count on wide experience, ranging from a tooth extraction to all kinds of general surgery.

When he had saved enough money for the trip he went to Vienna. At the University of Vienna Pathological Institute he worked with the man who had discovered the organism that causes meningitis, and also became an assistant to a noted pathologist. Then he went on to Munich to work with a prominent clinician. In those days young American doctors who sought to broaden their experience spent some time in one of the European medical centres just as artists went to Europe to study under the great masters.

After two years abroad Dr. Dick was ready to return to the United States. In 1910 he joined the McCormick Institute for Infectious Diseases where he began research work that led to his interest in scarlet fever. A year later he became Instructor in Pathology and Immunology at his alma mater. One of his students was Gladys Henry. She had come from even farther west, having been born in the same year as Dr. Dick, in Pawnee City, Nebraska. The postgraduate student in Dr. Dick's class was Dr. Henry with a medical degree she had earned at Johns Hopkins University. Early in 1914 teacher and student became husband and wife.

After a honeymoon in Europe, Dr. Gladys Dick took a post on the research staff of the McCormick Institute, while Dr. George Dick served as pathologist and director of laboratories in two Chicago hospitals. There he worked until the beginning of World War I. In 1917 he joined the Medical Corps, serving both in camps in the United States and in a Base Hospital overseas where he rose to the rank of Major. On his return from France, he decided that scarlet fever was the field in which he wanted most to work. The job that he had started some seven or eight years earlier needed finishing.

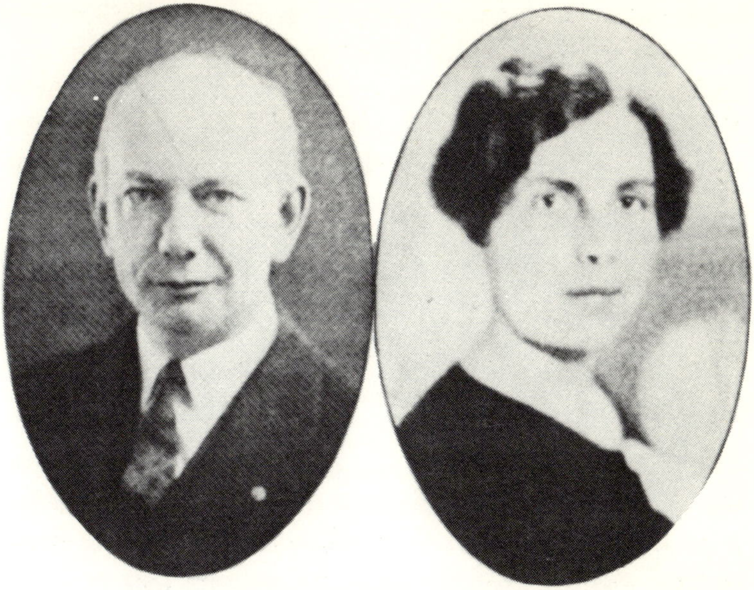

Drs. George F. and Gladys H. Dick

He joined his wife at the Institute, conducting research which he had to finance himself because there was no salary for him there. By practicing medicine and teaching at the University of Chicago, he was able to support his research.

What organism caused scarlet fever? There were several leads. Some thought it was a filterable virus, neither plant nor animal, too small to see, but capable of being carried from one person to another. Others thought it belonged to a class of bacteria called streptococci which, unlike bacilli, are little spheres instead of rods. The particular coccus which was usually seen in scarlet fever patients was the hemolytic streptococcus, so named because it destroyed red blood cells. But there were several types even of this one organism. Which one was the culprit? It was difficult to decide which type caused scarlet fever and which produced other diseases. Besides, it was possible that its presence in scarlet fever patients could mean that it was a casual invader, and not *the* cause of the disease.

This was the confused picture when the Dicks began their investigation, and it was what Dr. Dick meant when he said that even the first of Koch's requirements was lacking.

"Unless we are able to separate the particular organism from all others, we can't produce experimental scarlet fever," we can imagine the Dicks saying.

They began by taking swabs from throats, samples of blood, urine, and feces, skin scales from scarlet fever patients, and bits of organs from those who had died from the disastrous disease. With the material they thus gathered they prepared cultures in a variety of media. They found many colonies growing on their plates, but none more frequently than those of hemolytic streptococcus. This by itself proved nothing. They would have to separate the various bacteria they grew and inoculate, in turn, guinea pigs, rabbits, dogs, mice, pigeons, and small white pigs.

One by one they inoculated the stuff into the throat, squirted it under the skin, into the muscles and veins of their animals. We can almost see how, with the patience of a Koch, they tried to carry through the first steps—isolate the organism and reproduce the disease in an animal.

After two years they could report only that the animals occasionally developed a little fever, and once in a while a rash. But this wasn't scarlet fever. Besides, they got similar symptoms with a variety of organisms, and no one of them produced these signs consistently in any one species of animal.

They had to follow a new track. Collecting some blood from patients with scarlet fever, they separated the clear serum from the blood cells. Then they mixed some of each of their cultures with samples of serum, examining a drop of the mixture under the microscope. Their reasoning was simple. Serum from convalescing patients should contain antibodies against the particular microbe that caused the disease. It was known that active serum would cause the little spheres to clump, a process called agglutination. Only the microbes that caused the disease would clump into a knot with the active serum. Any others would remain unaffected. It was a test for separating the one "guilty" from all the "innocent" microbes.

Two more years went by in this detective work and the Dicks could report that the hemolytic streptococcus was the one organism that was most constantly clumped. It gave a *positive clumping test*. This was the clue to follow up through the next step.

They would try to produce scarlet fever. With the streptococcus cultures they obtained from blood, mucus, macerated scales, ground tonsils, and spleens directly after death of patients, they inoculated animals. But none of them contracted the disease. There was only one conclusion: animals were not susceptible; they couldn't contract this disease.

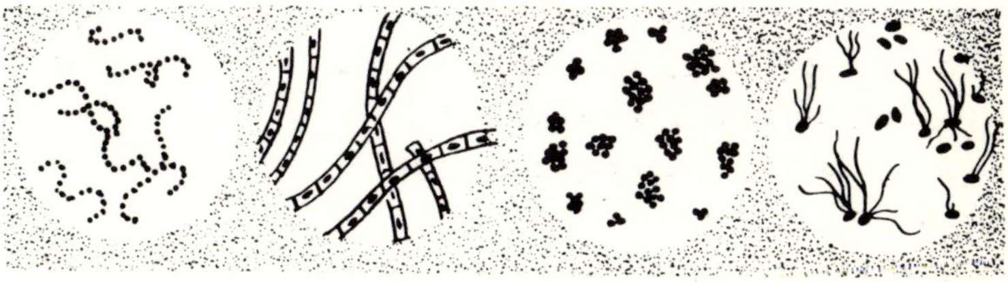

These bacteria cause (from left to right): scarlet fever, anthrax, boils, typhoid fever

"We will have to try human volunteers. That was what Jenner did, and found it successful," Drs. Dick must have decided.

It was necessary to produce the disease experimentally to prove that they had its cause. In their work on scarlet fever, Dr. Dick recalled forty years later, the most interesting thing that happened was the readiness with which people volunteered. "Contrary to our expectation that it would be hard to get such volunteers, we had offers from people in nearly all the States in the Union who offered to come to Chicago without any compensation to be inoculated," he wrote.

It wasn't easy sailing even after that, for it was difficult to produce the disease even in man. Less than half of the people contract the disease when they are exposed to it. Some older persons may have had it without its having been recognized; others may have a natural immunity.

Checking for the presence of the streptococcus and using the clumping test, they found that the scarlet fever microbe is seen in the throat mucus, but not in the blood, in early cases without any complications. This much they found out when they inoculated healthy young adults, who had not had the disease, with blood serum taken from patients with scarlet fever in the early stages. They swabbed the tonsils with the serum, and watched daily for signs of sore throat, fever, rash on the skin and palate. But the volunteers remained without a sign of disease. They next injected a bit of the serum under the skin, but again the results were negative. All this proved that in the early stage the organism was not in the bloodstream.

Was the cause after all a filterable virus? They inoculated their human "guinea pigs" with filtered material. Still they remained well. This was apparently not the path to follow. They would have to try pure cultures.

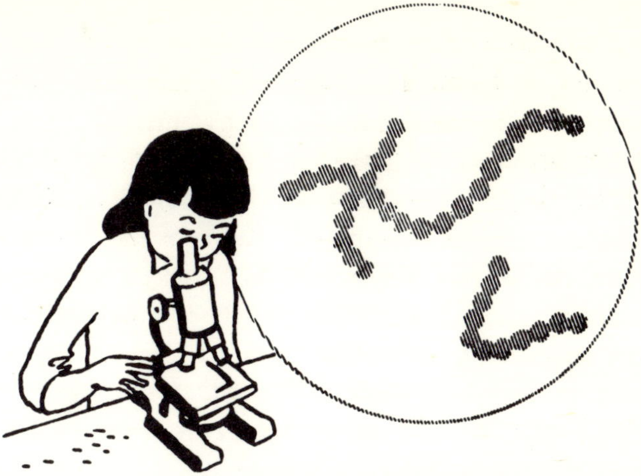

Different bacteria form groupings of different shapes. These chains are found in "strep" sore throat

Thirty volunteers were ready to undergo the test. The Dicks swabbed their throats with day-old cultures of hemolytic streptococcus obtained from the tonsils of scarlet fever patients. Some of the volunteers developed sore throats, swollen glands, but as yet no rash.

Then one day a nurse who was taking care of a patient with scarlet fever acquired the disease. Two days before the full-blown symptoms appeared, she noticed that she had a sore finger. When the rash was at its reddest, Dr. Dick obtained a bit of the pus from her finger and grew a culture of it on fresh sheep's blood agar. Translucent gray colonies, each about the size of a pinhead, grew on the agar. Surrounding each colony was a tiny rim in which the sheep's blood cells were destroyed. Each speck of a colony was a pure culture of hemolytic streptococcus!

This time they inoculated a group of volunteers with the pure cultures. One of five subjects developed all the symptoms of scarlet fever, her rash persisting for four weeks; by the end of that time the typical scaling of the skin was almost complete. At last they had produced scarlet fever artificially!

Dr. Dick himself got a mild scarletinal rash, but he and his wife were not yet sure of the cause. It could still be a filterable virus. They strained their culture through one of those fine filters that Roux and Yersin had used to separate the poison from the diphtheria bacillus. They swabbed the throats of their patient volunteers with the filtrate, and it seems strange to say that they remained disappointingly well.

Two weeks later they tried unfiltered cultures in the same subjects. This time, after 48 hours, one of them developed scarlet fever. This experiment furnished further evidence that the disease was not caused by a filterable virus. It must be due to the hemolytic streptococcus itself!

Then new difficulties arose in the search. There were at least two kinds of this bug. One strain, the one they recovered from the sick subject and grew in pure culture, could be identified by the particular food it fermented. Was scarlet fever produced by other "streps" that did not ferment this food? They would have to rule out that possibility.

Thus far, Dr. Dick could report, "All of Koch's laws were fulfilled, except that one which requires that the organism be constantly present in the disease." But they rarely found the organism in the blood. Perhaps this case was parallel to diphtheria. It was possible that the microbes grew in the throat, but manufactured something which, when it leaked into the blood, gave people the skin rash.

There was yet another lead they had to follow to its logical end. They recalled that back in 1916 when they had injected killed streptococcus into the skin, they noticed a "slight local redness that disappeared at the end of 48 hours." What was responsible for this reaction?

"If we could find this substance, it might be possible to use it in skin tests to determine which of our volunteers were susceptible to the disease." So they took some of the material that came through their fine filter, and had failed to produce the disease in their previous experiments, and injected a bit of it into the skin. Sure enough, there appeared a little red patch, but only in those subjects who never had the disease. Persons who were convalescing from scarlet fever failed to show the reaction. This discovery made their work so much easier. They could now sift their volunteer population.

Then they picked two volunteers: one with a positive skin reaction and one who failed to show the little red patch. The next step was to inoculate the first subject with the strain of organism that *didn't* ferment the special food, and he developed scarlet fever.

With full certainty, the doctors wrote: "The hemolytic streptococci used in these experiments had now fulfilled all the requirements of Koch's laws and the conclusion that they are the cause of scarlet fever was justified."

The filtrates from cultures of both strains produced the skin reactions in susceptible persons. They now pursued this clue. Mixing equal amounts of the toxic filtrate with serum taken from scarlet fever convalescents they tried yet another test. In one group of subjects with a positive skin reaction they injected the mixture, and in a similar group they used the toxin mixed with salt solution. One day later, the persons who received the mixture of toxin and convalescent serum showed no red spot, while those who had the blank salt solution with the toxin did get the telling red spot.

The convalescent serum must contain antitoxin! It provided a temporary protection to their susceptible subject.

Doctors Dick then embarked on a bolder venture: they would try to make susceptible persons immune. Using only those subjects who gave a positive Dick test, the red patch on the skin, they injected larger amounts of the toxic filtrate. Within a couple of days they developed fever, nausea, and finally also the typical scarlet fever rash. When they recovered, they no longer gave a positive skin reaction. Their blood had attained the power to neutralize the poison. They had become actively immune, having their own potent convalescent serum.

Together, these experiments showed that they were dealing with a specific substance capable of producing scarlet fever. It was a soluble toxic substance from the organism and not a filterable virus that was responsible for the disease. This substance was a true toxin capable of stimulating the tissues to produce antitoxin.

Dr. George and Gladys Dick were the first experimental team in the history of infectious disease to carry out the job from start to finish.

They found the cause of the disease, developed a skin test to find out who was susceptible, and found a way to protect those who might get it, and to cure those who had come down with it. Their experiments, running the gamut of discovering the cause, prevention, and cure, led to the final conquest of a disease which, though not extremely serious itself, leaves many with damaged hearts, kidneys, and other complications.

Then began the job of preventive immunization of all susceptible persons. When people "Dick-tested" positive, they could be protected from an attack of the full-blown disease!

After twelve years of research, the Dicks finished their job on scarlet fever. Dr. Gladys Dick continued with other work in the McCormick Institute of Infectious Diseases, while her husband went on with his practice and teaching. In the course of the years Dr. George became the head of the Department of Medicine at the Rush Medical College in Chicago, where he remained until his retirement. Prizes, awards, honorary degrees, and citations followed their momentous discovery. But the Dicks did not sit back. Even after retirement from active work, their interest in scarlet fever continued.

An intimate friend said that in spite of all their honours and their contributions in other areas of research, what they like most is to be remembered as "good doctors."

11

V-DAY IN POLIO WAR

THE END of our story is not about one man or even several; it is a tale of millions lined up against a disease—a crippler and killer they were determined to conquer. Their efforts have produced an effective vaccine against poliomyelitis.

The latest to be tackled, polio is by no means a new disease, for its history goes back at least 3000 years. Sculptured in a stone slab in ancient Egypt is the picture of a boy leaning on a crutch, one leg limp and helpless, and showing its shrunken muscles. Unknown to the sculptor, his faithful reproduction speaks to us across the ages—clearly the child was a polio victim.

Among the communicable maladies, even in the 1950s, polio actually ranks low as a cause of disease. There were many more cases of measles, scarlet fever, and whooping cough. Even in the most savage epidemics, it rarely struck more than 1 in every 1,000 of population. Yet the crippling paralysis which nearly always follows an attack made it one of the most feared diseases, and its near conquest one of the happiest achievements of our day.

The first to recognize polio or infantile paralysis as a distinct disease was Dr. Michael Underwood, a British physician, in

1784. Fifty years later, a German bone specialist, to whom a polio patient was brought, told the desperate mother that her boy was suffering not with a bone disease, but from something that damaged his nerve cells. Then in 1909, Dr. Karl Landsteiner, who is better known for his discovery of blood types, showed that polio was caused by an infectious agent. It could be transferred to monkeys from the ground-up spinal cord of children who died from the disease. By that time, several modern-time epidemics had taken their toll.

The first of these to occur in the United States was in 1894, in the valley of Otter Creek in the Green Mountains of Vermont. Child after child took sick with an upset stomach, high fever, headache, stiff neck, and sometimes convulsions. All too often, these symptoms were followed by paralysis and even death. More than a hundred children in Rutland and neighbouring villages succumbed before the baffled doctors, some of whom had never seen a case before, decided it was infantile paralysis.

Outbreaks in Sweden and other parts of Europe were being reported. In 1908, there were epidemics in the United States from New York to California, and one of the worst gripped New York in the summer of 1916. Panicked parents fled with their children or sent them to any place where they hoped they would be safe, even though there seemed to be no reason for its striking in one place rather than another. From then on, every summer came to be dreaded by parents as an annual menace. And even though some years brought fewer cases, on the whole polio was on the advance.

Strangely enough, the disease spread with great virulence in those parts of the world where sanitation was good, standards of hygiene high, and children were kept cleaner, better fed, and healthier. In the more primitive parts of the globe, epidemics were unknown. But when it was found that polio takes on many disguises the reason for this paradox was explained.

Millions of people who have had a sore throat, nausea, a headache or a "bad few days" have a "silent" infection with the polio virus. But if there was no paralysis the cases went unrecognized in perhaps 99 out of every 100 who had it. Yet it seems that this mild attack made them immune to a severe attack. The reason most people don't get it is that they "have had it," the authorities say.

It is now known that human beings are the great reservoir and transmitters of the polio virus. By natural exposure, babies become infected with the virus and develop protective antibodies in their blood. Perhaps four-fifths of us have had a mild unrecognized attack of the non-paralytic type of the disease and are protected. The rest are possible victims perhaps of the paralytic type during an epidemic. In crowded, poverty-ridden countries, however, most children by the age of two have had a "silent" infection. In the Near East, Central Africa, and the Orient, polio epidemics are rare. Blood samples from people in those regions show that they have acquired immunity from natural exposure.

The horrid disease is caused by a speck—the virus of poliomyelitis. Only the electron microscope reveals the fuzzy dot, so tiny that a million line up in one inch. But it takes only a few to paralyze and shrivel the muscles, arrest the rhythmic motion of the breathing muscles, and even to kill. It attacks young children most often, but adults are vulnerable too.

In the summer of 1921, it struck at a powerful, healthy man —Franklin Delano Roosevelt. At the age of 39, while vacationing on an island off the coast of New Brunswick, he was suddenly taken ill, and became paralyzed from the waist down.

The story of the conquest of polio is the tale of the courage, hard work, persistence, knowledge, and contribution of millions of people. Among these the late President Roosevelt has an honoured place.

Roosevelt had heard that swimming in the naturally warm waters at a former resort in Warm Springs, Georgia, strengthened the wasting muscles. He tried it first in 1924. Soon afterwards other polio patients came from all parts of the country to seek the reported improvement. Roosevelt then purchased the resort, financing the project called the Georgia Warm Springs Foundation, so that poor patients could also get the treatment.

Until he was elected president, he solicited funds for the maintenance of the sanatorium. His election to public office made the continuance of his work for the Foundation impossible. It was then that public-spirited citizens took over the task of collecting funds. The annual appeal which was named the "March of Dimes" by Eddie Cantor, the comedian, came to be known as the President's Birthday Celebration. The first was on January 30, 1934. Over a million dollars was collected annually in the March-of-Dimes, with Basil O'Connor, onetime law partner of Franklin D. Roosevelt, as its head. Four years later the National Foundation for Infantile Paralysis was organized. Its job was to plan and support the long battle ahead. A portion of its funds went to laboratories and hospitals for research that would lead to victory over polio.

Viruses are different from ordinary bacteria. For one thing, they are much smaller, but there are more important differences. The anthrax bacillus can live in the blood, grow, and reproduce. The diphtheria bacillus produces a toxin which poisons the blood. But like all other viruses, the poliovirus can only multiply inside living cells. Once it gets into a cell it takes control and directs the energy systems of the cell to producing more poliovirus. Eventually the cell is destroyed. If the cell involved is in the brain or spinal cord it cannot be replaced and if enough new cells are destroyed paralysis and even death follow. Because of the fact that viruses are so closely involved in the metabolism of the cell which they infect they are not susceptible to treatment with antibiotics such as the penicillins or tetracyclines as bacteria are.

For a long time it was not known how the polio virus entered the body, which made it difficult to prevent its spread. It hit the rich and the poor, those in the country and those in the city, mostly young but also adults. Epidemics occurred in the summer and early autumn, but isolated cases could appear at any time of the year. Was it spread by flies, water, milk, sewage, or dust? Many facts had to be gathered and much research was required before suitable defences against polio could be devised. In fact, the first vaccine, prepared twenty years before the Salk vaccine, failed tragically, causing paralysis and death in some. More had to be learned about the "nature of the beast" before it could be attacked. Progress was slow and the results more often discouraging than fruitful.

It wasn't until 1949 that a group of Harvard researchers broke through to a clear path. They found a way to grow polio virus in a test-tube, and not on nerve tissue. This was a big step forward. It was no longer necessary to depend upon monkeys in whose brains and spinal cords the polio virus flourished. The virus would grow on other tissues but thrived best on a bit of monkey's kidney tissue. Since it could be grown in a flask, much more of it would become available for hundreds of different kinds of experiments. But even more important, it explained the mystery of how the polio virus reached the nerves. It could enter through the mouth, be swallowed, start its growth in the cells of the intestine, and eventually get to the nerves. For their trail-blazing discovery the Harvard scientists—Dr. John F. Enders, Dr. Thomas Weller, and Dr. Frederick Robbins—received the Nobel Prize.

Two years later it was found that the little deadly speck was not one but triplets: "Brunhilde" (after a chimpanzee), "Lansing" (after the city where it was first identified), and "Leon" (after a young patient). There were three types of polio virus, and each type could produce all forms of the disease. A person may have become immune to the most prevalent Type I through a

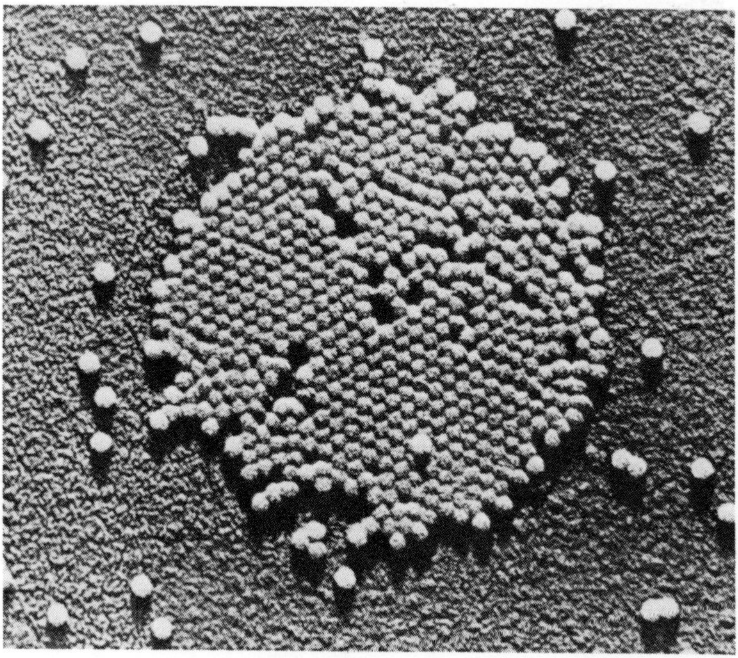

A strain of Type II poliomyelitis virus enlarged approximately 180,000 times under the electron microscope

"silent" infection, and still be struck by Type II or Type III. This discovery explained the failure of some early vaccines. An effective vaccine would have to be made from all three types of virus!

Then came a world-wide screening or typing of 100 strains to find the particular strains of each of the three types that caused polio. Research teams in several universities in the United States spent three years working with 30,000 monkeys to find the three culprits.

In 1952, an important discovery by Dr. Dorothy Horstmann of Yale and Dr. David Bodian of Johns Hopkins Medical School revealed the path of the virus to the vulnerable nerve cells. They found that in its journey to the cells it selected for attack, it travelled through the bloodstream. If it were possible to intercept it in the blood, it could be prevented from getting to the nerves. If antibodies could be built up in sufficient quantities in the blood, they would provide a defence against invasion of nerve centres. This was the blueprint for a defensive vaccine. But it would take time.

In the meantime, some scientists looked about for temporary defences. They thought of utilizing the immunity many adults have acquired from natural exposure to the disease. Such persons had built up antibodies which are carried by one of the blood proteins—gamma globulin, GG for short. Some people may have antibodies against Type I, and others against Type II or III. But if GG were collected from many persons, a pool of all three antibodies could be established. Borrowing GG from such a pool would be like making a loan to children who hadn't yet developed their own. It would, of course, be a borrowed immunity, lasting only five or six weeks.

GG worked. It saved some children from polio, and in others it weakened the attack. In 1952, a million doses were injected into children and pregnant women in epidemic areas. But GG was not the final answer. It wore off before the danger was entirely over and had to be given every summer. Also, who could know in advance which child would become a victim and, therefore, needed the protection? Besides, the GG pool was not big enough. A pint of human blood made only one shot. It was a delaying action, but not a sure defence.

The search for a vaccine had to go on.

One of the universities commissioned by the National Foundation to classify the 100 strains of viruses from every part of the world was the University of Pittsburgh. It fell to the lot of a thirty-five-year-old scientist who had been working with the influenza virus in the university's Virology laboratory to join in the "fingerprinting" job of the polio virus types. The slim, dark-haired, bespectacled student of viruses was Jonas Edward Salk.

Jonas Salk was a product of New York City's public education system. Born in Manhattan, in 1914, he was the eldest son of a dress manufacturer. A precocious pupil in his local school, Jonas was eligible for entrance into Townsend Harris High School which had been maintained for the studious, promising boys. In three, instead of four years these boys completed a much more rigorous high school curriculum than in the ordinary school. Salk graduated at sixteen from Townsend Harris, and at nineteen from the College of the City of New York. In high school he had planned to study law, and so he took no science courses until he entered college. It was only then that he got his first taste of science which became his life.

He chose medicine as a career and enrolled in New York University Medical School. Early in his medical studies he knew that he wanted to do research. In fact, after his freshman year he departed from the usual medical curriculum to work in protein chemistry for a year. By the time he completed his internship he had fully decided not to go into private practice. When people pointed out that research didn't pay as well as medical practice, he had a ready answer: there was more in life than money.

The National Research Council granted Salk a fellowship in virus research and he left New York to join one of his professors and sponsors who had taken a post in the University of Michigan, at Ann Arbor. There Salk worked until 1947, when the Dean of Pittsburgh's School of Medicine was looking about for a bright young man to head a new department. It was just about the time when those wonder drugs, the antibiotics, had cracked the defences of most bacterial infections. But they were useless against virus infections. The Pittsburgh dean was eager to chart a new path in the crusade against disease. His idea was to establish a Department of Virology, and Jonas Salk seemed to him to be the promising virologist. He was then on the trail of the influenza virus.

There were at first no elaborate plans for a well-equipped laboratory nor funds for a full staff for the new department. For Dr. Salk the removal to the basement laboratory in the Municipal Hospital connected with the university was a gamble. He was leaving Michigan for what might have turned out to be a dead end. But for a man who devotes sixteen hours of six days of every week to research, the glamour of a beautiful laboratory had little importance. There was only the big problem of virus diseases. So he, his wife, and their two sons went to the coal and steel metropolis.

Dr. Salk joined the quest for a polio vaccine when it became certain that all known strains of polio virus belonged to three main types. By this time his staff had increased, and together with them he typed three-fourths of the strains during a three-year project. To make an effective vaccine, there had to be plenty of virus; it had to be grown on non-nervous tissue to avoid possible damage to human nerves of virus grown on nerve tissue; a proper broth for growing the virus had to be selected; three types of virus had to be included in the vaccine and finally a way had to be found to kill or weaken the virus and still leave intact its power to stimulate the production of protective antibodies.

This was the blueprint for an effective vaccine which Dr. Salk sketched for himself. Dr. Ender's discovery that monkey kidney was a good virus-growing tissue was confirmed by his own experiments. Then he tested many media to find the one on which the virus flourished best, and selected one recipe—No. 199—that contained 62 ingredients, which had been developed in a Toronto laboratory for growing cancer cells.

He minced the kidney tissue and placed it in flasks. Then he added the nutrient broth which had the necessary ingredients for virus growth. Every few days fresh nutrient medium No. 199 was added, and the tissue culture tested for germs and viruses. Then one strain of a specific type of virus was added to the mixture. When enough virus attached itself to the tissue particles, the virus was "harvested." Again the liquid was tested for possible intruders—contaminating bacteria or other kinds of virus. Was the virus potent? Did it make guinea pigs and rabbits sick?

When live virus is injected into a living creature, it sets up immediate alarm signals. The body begins to manufacture protective antibodies. But active live virus couldn't be injected into children.

The next step was to kill the virus. The chemical chosen was formaldehyde which kills but at the same time preserves tissue from disintegration. Then followed a tedious process of trying dozens of concentrations of the chemical and different temperatures in which to bathe the virus culture—to kill it and yet have it retain the power to produce antibodies. How much culture would be needed to start the antibody manufacture? How much of the protective antibodies would be required for protection? Each of these questions had to be answered by injecting the killed virus into monkey tissue cells and into live animals.

By the middle of 1952 Dr. Salk was satisfied that he had answered these questions and that the vaccine could be tried in a human being. One had to be dead sure, however. Suppose the vaccine was not right! He decided to test it first in persons who had recovered from polio. They would have their own antibodies, but if the vaccine worked it should raise the antibody level—the *titer,* as it is called. If the vaccine proved active it would work like a booster shot, Dr. Salk reasoned. That is exactly what happened. The vaccine worked. It was then time to try it on people who were known not to have had the disease.

Vaccine that he developed in his own laboratory was shot into the first few children. In those days Dr. Salk didn't sleep very well, he acknowledged. Within a year and a half the confident but exacting Dr. Salk went into the community around Pittsburgh with his vaccine and needle, shooting it into adults and children, including his own (there were now three). It turned out to be completely safe: no bad reactions, no sore arms or fever in 1,000 cases. The titer reached the level he had hoped for. The children developed antibodies against all three types of virus. He measured it in their blood!

Dr. Salk was ready for a mass trial of the vaccine. But there were objections. Some said 1,000 cases were not enough to show

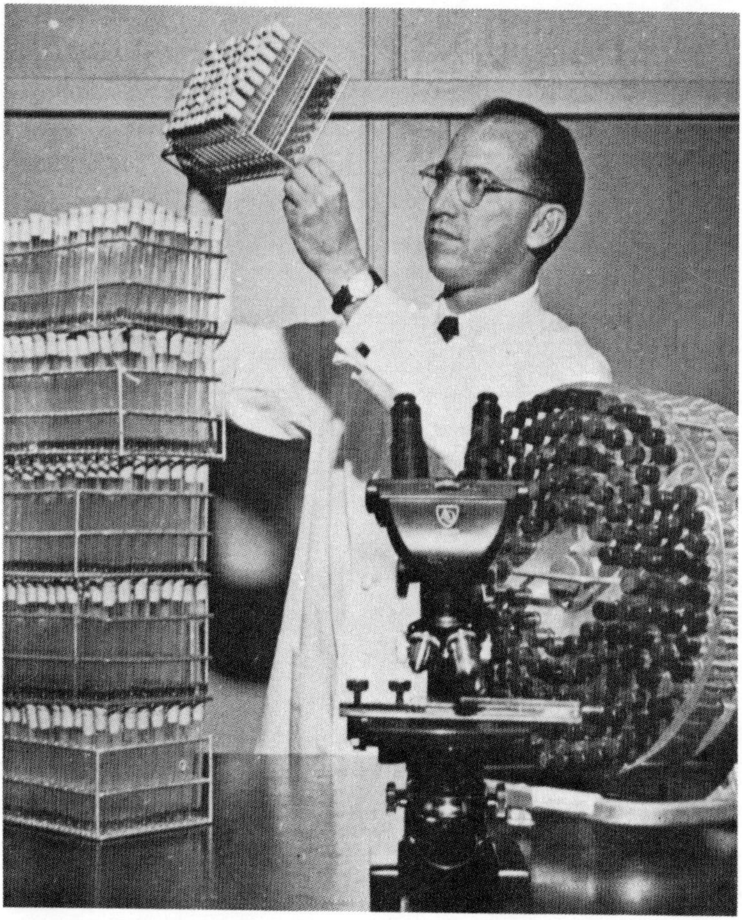

Dr. Jonas E. Salk checks tubes in colour test for antibodies

the safety of the vaccine. The doctor was in too much of a hurry, they insisted. There was also disagreement among the polio experts. Dr. Albert Sabin of Cincinnati argued that a killed-virus vaccine would not be as effective as a live-attenuated one. It would give immunity for perhaps only a year. People would be lulled into a false sense of security, he concluded.

Dr. Salk agreed to continue with his solo vaccinating programme, getting parents to consent to having their children receive the shots. Some had three shots, others only two or one, until within a few weeks he had raised his quota of preliminary trials to 7,000. But were these children protected against polio? This was still the big question that would be answered only during a polio epidemic.

In the spring of 1954 came the time for an important decision. Should mass trials be delayed for another year while more isolated trials were done, or did the scientists have the obligation to make available a useful vaccine immediately? This difficult decision was finally made by the National Foundation. The mass trials were to be begun in April, in time for the anticipated polio outbreaks in the South where the warm weather came earlier.

Dr. Thomas Francis, Jr., Dr. Salk's one-time professor, was chosen as the right man for the job; despite his fondness for his former student, he could be trusted to give impartial judgment. Dr. Francis undertook it on certain conditions: children in the first three classes would be inoculated; half would get the vaccine, and half would get some ordinary fluid. And nobody was to know who got which, until a year later, when he and his co-workers at the University of Michigan would decode the numbers. Only then would the results be made known.

The story is now part of history. The mammoth test was set in motion and 1,830,000 children took part, their parents hopefully giving permission. Salk vaccine was given to 440,000 children, most of whom received three shots, and 210,000 others received a dummy shot. Another 1,180,000 in the same towns and neighbourhoods received neither. They were the controls, without whom the test would not have been complete.

The children chosen for the test were five to nine years old. In eleven states, first, second, and third formers got the shots, half receiving the real thing, and the others the liquid that looked the same, but had no vaccine. In another 33 states, vaccine was inoculated into second-form pupils only, while third-form children were the controls.

So much vaccine was required for this giant project that it couldn't be manufactured in a university laboratory. Commercial drug manufacturers went to work. The vaccine was triple-tested by the companies, the U. S. Public Health Service, and by Dr. Salk's laboratory.

On April 26, 1954, the crucial human test was begun. Classrooms were hastily converted into test stations where teachers, parents, the milkman, and the mayor offered their services to the army of youngsters who were lined up to receive their shots. Some came to entertain the waiting boys and girls, others to bring lollipops as consolation, but all helped in a vast national project.

Twenty thousand physicians and health officers, twice as many nurses, thousands of teachers, and nearly a quarter of a million other citizens volunteered to help carry out the programme. Even children were donors—donors of blood samples for testing the presence of antibodies. Proudly they wore their Polio Pioneer buttons and Certificates of Bravery.

By the beginning of the summer the "shooting" stage of the test was over. Then came the tally, the checking of what happened to the children. Did any of them get polio? What kind? Were there any deaths? The statisticians, the scientific "bookkeepers," went to work to examine and chart the thousands of facts that were gathered in the field and sent to the Polio Evaluation Center at the University of Michigan. Dr. Francis of the university's School of Public Health directed the sifting of the information that flowed from the mail trucks into his office. Nearly 150 million pieces of information had to be gone over. From these facts would come the answer as to whether the vaccine worked.

As the day approached when the answer would be given, there was wild guessing, prediction, speculation, and mounting excitement. Drug companies went into high-gear production, building up the supply of vaccine, should the green light be given by Dr. Francis who held the key to the great secret.

On the morning of April 12, 1955, Dr. Francis was ready to disclose the results of the immense field trial. An enormous volume representing the work of thousands of statisticians, physicians, and technicians contained the findings of the year's study.

As Dr. Francis was about to make the official announcement, the hushed excitement in Rackham Hall on the Michigan campus reached a climactic pitch. THE MASS TESTS SHOW THAT THE SALK VACCINE WAS 60 TO 90 PER CENT EFFECTIVE.

Over six times as many more of the unvaccinated children were paralyzed by polio, than among the vaccinated. One hundred thirteen of the protected children, and 750 of the unvaccinated were taken sick with polio. There was not a single death among the vaccinated group, while 15 deaths occurred in the unvaccinated. The injections themselves produced no severe reactions and *no polio*. The vaccine was safe and effective in 80 to 90 of 100 children.

As the chief hero of the occasion rose to speak, his words were lost in thunderous applause. Dr. Jonas E. Salk presented recommendations about timing and "priming" of inoculations. But the typewriters were already clicking out the telephoned messages of victory. Throughout the world hearts were gladdened.

Tributes to Dr. Salk were pouring in: a citation from President Eisenhower; a proposal that Salk be given a special Congressional Medal of Honour; and a bill in the U. S. Senate that $10,000 should be added to his salary as university professor. Salk funds for further research were being started in all parts of the country.

Within a few days after the announcement that the Salk polio vaccine was "safe, potent, effective," children trooped into line to receive the first shots of vaccine in a programme arranged for by the Foundation. Within a week four million doses had been shipped to health officers to build up the defences against an anticipated summer attack of polio. But just as it seemed that the new vaccine was closing in on polio, there was a tragic setback in the campaign.

At the end of April came the alarming news that polio had developed in a number of children who had been inoculated. The vaccine was traced in every instance to one firm that had been licensed to produce it. Something had gone wrong! Further distribution from the particular drug company was stopped, and the vaccine that had already gone out was recalled. As the number of reported cases began to mount, an investigation by experts was in full swing, and all further inoculations were ordered stopped by the U. S. Public Health Service, until the trouble was found. When the report finally came in, it was discovered that in six of nine lots of vaccine there was live virus. Eleven persons had died and 200 had developed polio. Some of these had been inoculated with vaccine from these lots, and the rest were members of the families where the accident had occurred.

More rigid safety tests were instituted. The vaccine had to be filtered within three days before the chemical treatment with formaldehyde was begun. The chemical cooking was extended for an additional three days. A fixed amount of each vaccine batch had to be tested for live virus particles. Before shipping, the bottled vaccine was to be tested once more. After pooling the batches of each type of virus, a large sample was again tried on monkey kidney cells and injected into the brain and spinal cord of monkeys. These additional precautions helped to restore confidence that was very nearly shattered by the mishap.

Then came more confusion in the administration of the programme. There wasn't enough vaccine to go around. Parents were frantically anxious to protect their children, and those most vulnerable to an attack were often the last to receive the vaccine. Despite the debates, the misadministration and criticism of the programme, millions of children were vaccinated through the summer, and the Salk vaccine went through its next great test. It was saving children from paralytic polio. There was much less polio among the vaccinated children in areas where epidemics raged. In 1956 the inoculation programme was back "on the track" as the supplies of vaccine caught up with the need.

In Britain plans had been made to carry out a controlled trial in 1955 when news of the vaccine-associated cases broke. The trial was postponed for a year and the vaccine finally used in 1956 and licensed in the U. K. in 1957 contained a different strain of Type I poliovirus from that used in the U. S. A.

Meanwhile in another approach to the problem two other groups of workers were attempting to develop live vaccines

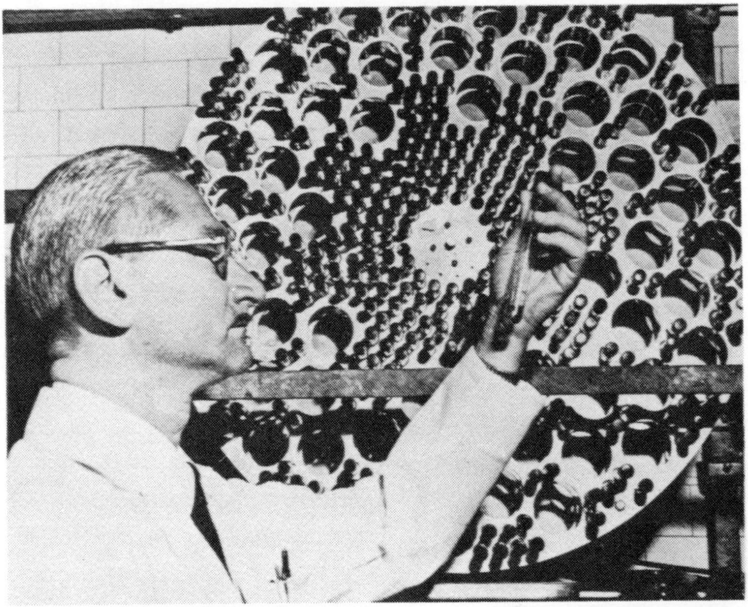

Dr. Albert E. Sabin. Can a vaccine be made with living but "tame" virus?

against polio. The idea was that these should consist of weakened strains of the three types of virus, which would produce infection only in the intestine. This should, argued Dr. Sabin of Cincinnati and Drs. Cox and Koprowski of the Lederle Laboratories at Pearl River, mimic the natural infection, but would not spread into the blood stream and therefore could not get to the nervous system and produce paralysis. They further argued that these attenuated viruses would give a better and more lasting protection than Salk's killed vaccine as they would stimulate local resistance in the gut as well as antibody which would be present in the blood.

They had the additional attraction that they could be given by mouth and did not need to subject the recipients to a series of injections by needle.

In the war on polio, Dr. Sabin was perhaps the earliest battler. A doctor with a bent for research, Albert Bruce Sabin saw in science a way to help people. He was born in Byalostock, in 1906. In 1921, the Sabin family left behind the anti-Semitism in Poland and came to settle in the United States. While the older members of the family were still in the throes of establishing themselves in a new homeland, the boy, eager to become Americanized, quickly mastered the English language and graduated from a New Jersey high school within two years.

At first it seemed that Albert would not have the opportunity for further study, because his parents were too poor to send him to college. But a relative who had helped to bring the family to the United States now invited Albert to come to New York, offering to pay for his tuition through dental school. After two years of dental training, Sabin suddenly changed his course. Reading about the exciting achievements of science heroes in the battle against disease-producing microbes, he decided to take the path of medicine and research.

In this new career he received his inspiration from Dr. William H. Park, a famous bacteriologist and public health leader. To young Sabin, Dr. Park was what Dr. Francis was to Salk. Sabin worked his way through college, then went on to the School of Medicine at New York University, where Dr.

Park was Professor of Bacteriology. In a corner of his laboratory, Professor Park started the earnest young student on a project in bacteriology. When he graduated from medical school in 1931, Sabin began work on a problem in polio suggested to him by Dr. Park.

The results of Sabin's early work were disappointing, but he kept on. In 1936, in the laboratories of the Rockefeller Institute, he found that the polio virus could be made to grow in the test tube—on nerve tissue removed from the body. This was a tremendous forward stride, for now he could undertake to breed generations of ever weaker strains of the virus. From then on for twenty years he followed his goal: taking the sting out of the invisible enemy.

Three years later Sabin scored another major victory. It was in Cincinnati's University College of Medicine that he and his team tracked down the virus to the intestinal tract in man. He found that this is where the polio virus lived mainly, but it had the power also to deal a paralyzing and deadly blow to the nervous system. If the paralytic polio virus strain could be weakened sufficiently, it could perhaps be made harmless to nerves. At the same time its growth in the intestine would goad the tissues into building antibodies. This was the reasoning behind the virus tamer's job of "domestication" of the deadly particles.

The Cincinnati team went into full swing after Dr. Enders' breakthrough which made possible the growing of the polio virus in non-nervous tissue.

They snipped bits of monkey kidney and added an enzyme to the flask to dissolve the connective tissue, leaving only the living kidney cells. They fed these cells a special diet to keep them alive. Viruses are finicky eaters—they grow only on live cells. Then began a series of transfers of the virus from one kidney culture to another—30, 40, 100 times. After many such passages the virus lost its sting. When finally it was injected into monkeys' brains, it had become harmless. If harmless to monkeys, perhaps also to people, the scientists reasoned.

Dr. Ramos Alvarez of the Sabin team discovered that Mexican children were especially resistant to Type I virus. He and Dr. Sabin boarded the first plane to Mexico City and began to collect swabs from the intestines of normal healthy children who had been in contact with polio. The samples obtained from these rectal swabs were placed into test tubes with monkey kidney cells, and were flown back to the laboratory in Cincinnati.

Side by side with the collection of virus tamed by nature in healthy, robust children, the process of patient taming in the laboratory went on. Both kinds of weakened virus were harmless to animals; and so the daring yet cautious inoculation of human beings began. First the scientists tried it on themselves, swallowing the virus in milk. The results were the same as if they had contracted a "silent" infection naturally. Their bodies were building antibody defenses to polio.

The ways of taming are indeed ingenious. Dr. Koprowski started on still another trail. He began with a deadly virus derived originally from a British soldier who died of polio during World War II. First he injected the Type II virus into the brain of a mouse. A gram of this virus would kill 1,000 mice. From the brain of the first mouse that died he extracted the virus and passed it on to the next and to a third. After many such passages the virus became more toxic to mice, so that a gram would now kill 10 million mice. More potent for mice, it became less potent in other animals—hamsters and monkeys. It was tamed by being "trained away" from monkeys and men.

Then he tried to establish the virus in fertile hens' eggs—

still farther away from human beings. The virus at first would not accommodate itself to its new host. But after passage through 115 generations of hamsters it grew in eggs! With a tiny dental drill a hole was made in scores of eggs into which a little of the virus was dropped. The hole was sealed with paraffin, and in this shell-encased home the virus propagated in the incubator. Again it was passed from egg to egg, and periodically tested on monkeys. After 100 passages it lost its sting for monkeys; it hardly made them sick. Yet it forced the monkeys' tissues to produce antibodies to Type II strains.

Even before this work of taming polio virus in hens' eggs was completed, a feeble-minded boy in a state institution was

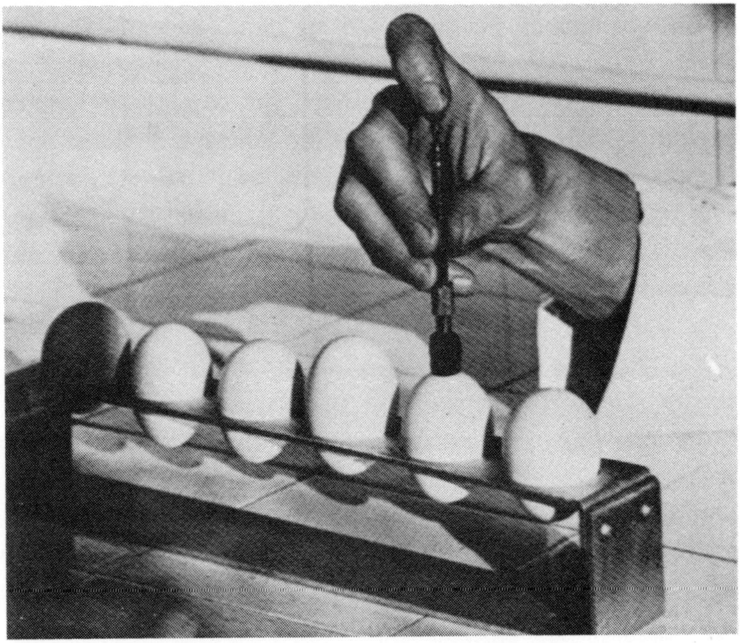

Inoculation of eggs at the Pasteur Institute in Paris

fed tamed virus in 1950. So that millions of others might some day be protected against polio, his parents consented to this test with their luckless child. This first child to swallow a spoonful of live virus in chocolate milk is still alive today, without having succumbed to polio!

At the same time Sabin went on to develop a strain of virus that would multiply in the intestinal tract. In 1953 he had his first triumph. He had bred particles of formerly paralytic virus that no longer produced paralysis even when he shot them directly into the brains of monkeys and chimpanzees. These new strains when fed in large amounts to chimpanzees grew in their intestines. The next step was to feed the virus to human beings. First Sabin himself, then his co-workers, swallowed the cultures of altered virus.

Soon volunteers in the prison of the U. S. Industrial Reformatory at Chillicothe, Ohio joined in the experiments. The breeding of a safe live virus continued for two more years until in 1956 Dr. Sabin was satisfied that his wife and children could be protected against paralytic polio by swallowing the tamed virus. Then the Soviet Union, whose scientists were working along the same lines, decided to put the Sabin vaccine into mass trials.

In June 1959, the International Scientific Congress on Live Virus met in Georgetown University in Washington. Dr. Sabin announced that live polio virus had been safely given to four-and-a-half million persons in large-scale tests in Mexico, Malaya, the Soviet Union, Poland, and Czechoslovakia. The meeting was sponsored by the World Health Organization, the Pan-American Health Organization, and the Sister Kenny Foundation. The purpose was to evaluate a world-wide program to banish polio. By 1960 close to 12 million children had received the Sabin live virus vaccine by mouth and in 1961 it was brought into use in Britain and the United States.

Since that time hundreds of millions of children all over the world have been protected by Sabin vaccine and its effectiveness in wiping out the dread of polio is clear from the health data from all the countries where it has been used. In the U. S. A. the number of cases of paralytic polio had fallen from 18,308 in 1954 to 17 in 1971 and in England and Wales from a 1955 figure of 3,712 to one of 6 in 1971.

But the battle is still not completely won. When a disease is brought under control to such an extent, people rapidly forget its dangers and many young parents today who have never known the horror of a polio epidemic neglect to have their children vaccinated. This has been reflected in an increase in the number of cases occurring in the past two years in some countries where the percentage of children vaccinated has shown a decline. Polio could come back if vaccination against it is neglected, and there are still many tropical and subtropical countries where it is still a problem and from which infection could be carried either by immigrants or returning holiday makers.

Virus grew in intestines so could be taken by mouth & would give immunity.

FROM JENNER TO SALK AND SABIN

In man's war against his unseen enemies many glorious battles have been won. Diphtheria and smallpox are scourges of the past. Many younger doctors have never seen a case of typhoid or yellow fever. The Sauer vaccine has taken the "whoop" out of whooping cough, and gamma globulin tides a child over the early years when measles may be dangerous. Rabies is no longer invulnerable and tetanus can be prevented by a shot in time.

At six months old a baby receives a triple inoculation against diphtheria, whooping cough and tetanus, and an oral dose of anti-polio vaccine. A booster dose against these diseases is given at five years, omitting that against whooping cough, to strengthen the child's defences before starting school. An inoculation against measles is given between one and two years of age, and one against rubella between eleven and fourteen years. A BCG injection is given at thirteen years, and a booster shot against polio and tetanus to school-leavers.

Pasteur's great dream of the conquest of childhood infections is fast coming true. No longer do they throw such dire fear into parents, for in the last decade, deaths from these causes have been reduced by 80 per cent.

Some virus diseases still challenge our ingenuity, but on the road to final victory, man has marched a long way from Jenner to Salk and Sabin.

INDEX

INDEX